Toxin and Immunotoxin Based Therapeutic Approaches

Toxin and Immunotoxin Based Therapeutic Approaches

Editors

Massimo Bortolotti
Letizia Polito
Andrea Bolognesi

MDPI • Basel • Beijing • Wuhan • Barcelona • Belgrade • Manchester • Tokyo • Cluj • Tianjin

Editors
Massimo Bortolotti
University of Bologna
Italy

Letizia Polito
University of Bologna
Italy

Andrea Bolognesi
University of Bologna
Italy

Editorial Office
MDPI
St. Alban-Anlage 66
4052 Basel, Switzerland

This is a reprint of articles from the Special Issue published online in the open access journal *Toxins* (ISSN 2072-6651) (available at: https://www.mdpi.com/journal/toxins/special_issues/Immunotoxin_Therapeutic).

For citation purposes, cite each article independently as indicated on the article page online and as indicated below:

LastName, A.A.; LastName, B.B.; LastName, C.C. Article Title. *Journal Name* **Year**, *Volume Number*, Page Range.

ISBN 978-3-0365-3064-2 (Hbk)
ISBN 978-3-0365-3065-9 (PDF)

Contents

About the Editors . . . . **vii**

Massimo Bortolotti, Letizia Polito and Andrea Bolognesi
Toxin and Immunotoxin Based Therapeutic Approaches
Reprinted from: *Toxins* **2022**, *14*, 63, doi:10.3390/toxins14010063 . . . . **1**

Yasser Hassan, Sherry Ogg and Hui Ge
Novel Binding Mechanisms of Fusion Broad Range Anti-Infective Protein Ricin A Chain Mutant-Pokeweed Antiviral Protein 1 (RTAM-PAP1) against SARS-CoV-2 Key Proteins in Silico
Reprinted from: *Toxins* **2020**, *12*, 602, doi:10.3390/toxins12090602 . . . . **5**

Shusei Hamamichi, Takeshi Fukuhara and Nobutaka Hattori
Immunotoxin Screening System: A Rapid and Direct Approach to Obtain Functional Antibodies with Internalization Capacities
Reprinted from: *Toxins* **2020**, *12*, 658, doi:10.3390/toxins12100658 . . . . **15**

Rosario Iglesias, Letizia Polito, Massimo Bortolotti, Manuela Pedrazzi, Lucía Citores, José M. Ferreras and Andrea Bolognesi
Primary Sequence and 3D Structure Prediction of the Plant Toxin Stenodactylin
Reprinted from: *Toxins* **2020**, *12*, 538, doi:10.3390/toxins12090538 . . . . **31**

Alexandra Fischer, Isis Wolf, Hendrik Fuchs, Anie Priscilla Masilamani and Philipp Wolf
Pseudomonas Exotoxin A Based Toxins Targeting Epidermal Growth Factor Receptor for the Treatment of Prostate Cancer
Reprinted from: *Toxins* **2020**, *12*, 753, doi:10.3390/toxins12120753 . . . . **49**

Rossella Rotondo, Sara Ragucci, Salvatore Castaldo, Maria Antonietta Oliva, Nicola Landi, Paolo V. Pedone, Antonietta Arcella and Antimo Di Maro
Cytotoxicity Effect of Quinoin, Type 1 Ribosome-Inactivating Protein from Quinoa Seeds, on Glioblastoma Cells
Reprinted from: *Toxins* **2021**, *13*, 684, doi:10.3390/toxins13100684 . . . . **63**

Hamid Hashemi Yeganeh, Mohammad Heiat, Marek Kieliszek, Seyed Moayed Alavian and Ehsan Rezaie
DT389-YP7, a Recombinant Immunotoxin against Glypican-3 That Inhibits Hepatocellular Cancer Cells: An In Vitro Study
Reprinted from: *Toxins* **2021**, *13*, 749, doi:10.3390/toxins13110749 . . . . **79**

Stefania Maiello, Rosario Iglesias, Letizia Polito, Lucía Citores, Massimo Bortolotti, José M. Ferreras and Andrea Bolognesi
Sequence, Structure, and Binding Site Analysis of Kirkiin in Comparison with Ricin and Other Type 2 RIPs
Reprinted from: *Toxins* **2021**, *13*, 862, doi:10.3390/toxins13120862 . . . . **97**

About the Editors

Massimo Bortolotti (PhD): Master degree in Pharmaceutical Chemistry. Researcher at the Laboratory of Toxic Enzyme and Immunotargeting, Department of Experimental, Diagnostic and Specialty Medicine (DIMES), University of Bologna.

Letizia Polito (Prof., PhD): Assistant Professor of General Pathology and Pathophysiology at the School of Medicine; Laboratory of Toxic Enzyme and Immunotargeting, Department of Experimental, Diagnostic and Specialty Medicine (DIMES), University of Bologna.

Andrea Bolognesi (Prof., PhD): Associate Professor of General Pathology and Pathophysiology at the School of Medicine; Laboratory of Toxic Enzyme and Immunotargeting, Department of Experimental, Diagnostic and Specialty Medicine (DIMES), University of Bologna.

toxins

Editorial

Toxin and Immunotoxin Based Therapeutic Approaches

Massimo Bortolotti *,†, Letizia Polito *,† and Andrea Bolognesi *,†

Department of Experimental, Diagnostic and Specialty Medicine—DIMES, Alma Mater Studiorum—University of Bologna, Via S. Giacomo 14, 40126 Bologna, Italy
* Correspondence: massimo.bortolotti2@unibo.it (M.B.); letizia.polito@unibo.it (L.P.); andrea.bolognesi@unibo.it (A.B.)
† These authors contributed equally to this work.

The concept of "magic bullets", i.e., drugs able to selectively act on target cells, formulated by Paul Ehrlich more than one century ago, gave rise to the idea of immunotargeting, one of the most studied approaches being based on antibodies carrying toxic moieties [1]. Bacterial or plant toxins can be joined to specific carriers through chemical linking or genetic engineering, antibodies being the most used carriers and the generated hybrid molecules having been named immunotoxins. These conjugates are functionally designed to eliminate pathological cells, finding applications in several fields such as cancer, immunological diseases or pain control.

Among plant toxins, the most used are ribosome-inactivating proteins (RIPs), a family of enzymes widely spread in the plant kingdom [2]. RIPs possess polynucleotide:adenosine glycosylase activity with the ability to remove adenines from several polynucleotide substrates, causing cell death. Adenine removal from *r*RNA, the first RIP activity to be described, damages ribosomes in an irreversible manner, causing the inhibition of protein synthesis; thus, explaining the origin of these proteins' name. RIPs are mainly classified as type 1, consisting of a single-chain protein with enzymatic activity, and type 2, consisting of an enzymatic A chain linked by a disulfide bond to a lectin B chain that is able to bind sugar-containing receptors on the cell membrane. The presence of the B chain in type 2 RIPs allows for a more rapid and efficient internalization into the cell than type 1 RIPs. For this reason, type 2 RIPs are highly cytotoxic [2]. Ricin is the most widespread and well-known type 2 RIP and also the most used in the construction of immunotoxins [3]. As RIPs have different intracellular substrates and are able to elicit more than one cell death pathway, they are drugs potentially suitable for a targeted cancer treatment. Furthermore, no drug resistance against toxins has been reported so far.

Among bacterial toxins, the most used are pseudomonas exotoxin A and the diphtheria toxin, which inhibit translation through the NAD-dependent ADP-ribosylation of the elongation factor-2, causing cell death [4]. Several immunotoxins have been developed using bacterial toxins and a variety of carriers specific for different targets. Up to date, three of these conjugates have been approved by the U.S. Food and Drug Administration for hematological cancer therapy [5].

The collection of seven scientific articles composing this Special Issue highlights the progress in the knowledge of toxins and immunotoxins; thus, underlying their potential in anticancer therapy.

In this Special Issue, a review article is included concerning the application of a new cell-based IT screening system offering several advantages in the formulation of new immunotoxins by enabling the straightforward and rapid selection of novel functional antibodies [6].

A fundamental requirement for the therapeutic application of toxins and their conjugates is the knowledge of their biochemical and structural properties, as well as of their binding, uptake, intracellular routing and substrate specificities. In this Special Issue, the complete amino acid sequence and 3D structure prediction of two potent type 2 Adenia

Citation: Bortolotti, M.; Polito, L.; Bolognesi, A. Toxin and Immunotoxin Based Therapeutic Approaches. *Toxins* **2022**, *14*, 63. https://doi.org/10.3390/toxins14010063

Received: 13 December 2021
Accepted: 12 January 2022
Published: 17 January 2022

Publisher's Note: MDPI stays neutral with regard to jurisdictional claims in published maps and institutional affiliations.

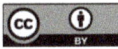

RIPs, namely, stenodactylin [7] and kirkiin [8], are determined. RIPs purified from the Adenia genus are known to be among the most lethal plant toxins [9]. The authors observed high structural and amino acid sequence homologies with other type 2 RIPs and particularly with those identified in plants belonging to the Adenia genus. The stenodactylin B chain showed a high degree of identity with B chains of other type 2 RIPs, supporting the hypothesis that the B chain is a product of a gene duplication event. A hemagglutination analysis revealed that both kirkiin and stenodactylin have similar affinities for D-galactose and lactose, although the affinity of kirkiin for these sugars was lower with respect to ricin. In both Adenia toxins, the replacement of histidine instead of ricin tyrosine in the sugar binding site of B chains was detected, possibly justifying the reduction in the sugar-binding affinity, although not seeming to affect cytotoxicity. Moreover, the cytotoxicity of quinoin, a recently purified type 1 RIP from quinoa seeds, was evaluated using human glioblastoma cell lines, and was seen to strongly reduce glioblastoma cell growth at concentrations in the nM range. Interestingly, an additive effect was found in primary cells treated with quinoin in combination with the chemotherapeutic temozolomide [10].

The Special Issue also focuses on the possibility to obtain selective and potent toxin-based conjugates able to be used for pharmacological purposes for different targets, with three interesting articles having been published in this regard. A fusion protein between the ricin A chain and pokeweed antiviral protein (RTAM-PAP1) was studied in silico for docking against various key proteins of SARS-CoV-2. The experiments revealed novel binding mechanisms of RTAM-PAP1 with a high affinity to numerous SARS-CoV-2 key proteins. RTAM-PAP1 was further characterized in a preliminary toxicity study in mice, and was found to be a potential therapeutic candidate [11]. The immunotoxin DT389-YP7 was obtained by fusing a truncated diphtheria toxin without a binding domain with a humanized YP7 scFv specific for a highly expressed Glypican-3 antigen on the surface of hepatocarcinoma cells, resulting specifically cytotoxic on the target HepG2 cell line. Cellular morphological changes, cell cycle arrest at the G2 phase, augment in radical oxygen species production, induction of apoptosis, and inhibition of cell movement were observed after the immunotoxin treatment [12]. The two recombinant anti epidermal growth factor receptor (EGFR) conjugates, EGF-PE40 and EGF-PE24mut, were constructed by fusing the epidermal growth factor (EGF) to PE40, which is the natural toxin domain of pseudomonas exotoxin A, or to PE24mut, its de-immunized variant. In EGFR-expressing prostate carcinoma cells, both conjugates inhibited protein synthesis and induced apoptosis in a concentration- and time-dependent manner, with IC_{50} values in the nanomolar/picomolar range. Interestingly, both conjugates were 600–140,000-fold more cytotoxic than the EGFR inhibitor erlotinib [13].

In conclusion, the studies collected in this Special Issue confirm the efficacy and the potentiality of toxins as payloads of immunotoxins/conjugates designed for targeted therapy on several cancer models. Moreover, the knowledge of the structural and binding characteristics of toxins and related conjugates, together with the elucidation of their mechanism(s) of action, provide useful information for better pharmacological strategies with the aim of achieving a higher specificity and potency in targeting and destroying cancer cells.

Author Contributions: M.B. wrote the editorial and gave a substantial and intellectual contribution to the work; L.P. organized and wrote the editorial, gave a substantial and intellectual contribution to the work; A.B. organized and gave a substantial and intellectual contribution to the work and revised the drafts and final version. All authors have read and agreed to the published version of the manuscript.

Funding: This paper was supported by RFO fund (Ricerca Fondamentale Orientata) for selected topics from the Alma Mater Studiorum, University of Bologna, by the Pallotti Legacies for Cancer Research and by Fondazione CARISBO, Project 2019.0539.

Informed Consent Statement: Not applicable.

Conflicts of Interest: The authors declare no conflict of interest.

References

1. Polito, L.; Djemil, A.; Bortolotti, M. Plant Toxin-Based Immunotoxins for Cancer Therapy: A Short Overview. *Biomedicines* **2016**, *4*, 12. [CrossRef]
2. Bolognesi, A.; Bortolotti, M.; Maiello, S.; Battelli, M.G.; Polito, L. Ribosome-Inactivating Proteins from Plants: A Historical Overview. *Molecules* **2016**, *21*, 1627. [CrossRef]
3. Polito, L.; Bortolotti, M.; Battelli, M.G.; Calafato, G.; Bolognesi, A. Ricin: An Ancient Story for a Timeless Plant Toxin. *Toxins* **2019**, *11*, 324. [CrossRef]
4. Akbari, B.; Farajnia, S.; Ahdi Khosroshahi, S.; Safari, F.; Yousefi, M.; Dariushnejad, H.; Rahbarnia, L. Immunotoxins in cancer therapy: Review and update. *Int. Rev. Immunol.* **2017**, *36*, 207–219. [CrossRef] [PubMed]
5. Havaei, S.M.; Aucoin, M.G.; Jahanian-Najafabadi, A. Pseudomonas Exotoxin-Based Immunotoxins: Over Three Decades of Efforts on Targeting Cancer Cells with the Toxin. *Front. Oncol.* **2021**, *11*, 781800. [CrossRef] [PubMed]
6. Hamamichi, S.; Fukuhara, T.; Hattori, N. Immunotoxin Screening System: A Rapid and Direct Approach to Obtain Functional Antibodies with Internalization Capacities. *Toxins* **2020**, *12*, 658. [CrossRef] [PubMed]
7. Iglesias, R.; Polito, L.; Bortolotti, M.; Pedrazzi, M.; Citores, L.; Ferreras, J.M.; Bolognesi, A. Primary Sequence and 3D Structure Prediction of the Plant Toxin Stenodactylin. *Toxins* **2020**, *12*, 538. [CrossRef] [PubMed]
8. Maiello, S.; Iglesias, R.; Polito, L.; Citores, L.; Bortolotti, M.; Ferreras, J.M.; Bolognesi, A. Sequence, Structure, and Binding Site Analysis of Kirkiin in Comparison with Ricin and Other Type 2 RIPs. *Toxins* **2021**, *13*, 862. [CrossRef] [PubMed]
9. Stirpe, F.; Bolognesi, A.; Bortolotti, M.; Farini, V.; Lubelli, C.; Pelosi, E.; Polito, L.; Dozza, B.; Strocchi, P.; Chambery, A.; et al. Characterization of highly toxic type 2 ribosome-inactivating proteins from *Adenia lanceolata* and *Adenia stenodactyla* (Passifloraceae). *Toxicon* **2007**, *50*, 94–105. [CrossRef] [PubMed]
10. Rotondo, R.; Ragucci, S.; Castaldo, S.; Oliva, M.A.; Landi, N.; Pedone, P.V.; Arcella, A.; Di Maro, A. Cytotoxicity Effect of Quinoin, Type 1 Ribosome-Inactivating Protein from Quinoa Seeds, on Glioblastoma Cells. *Toxins* **2021**, *13*, 684. [CrossRef] [PubMed]
11. Hassan, Y.; Ogg, S.; Ge, H. Novel Binding Mechanisms of Fusion Broad Range Anti-Infective Protein Ricin A Chain Mutant-Pokeweed Antiviral Protein 1 (RTAM-PAP1) against SARS-CoV-2 Key Proteins in Silico. *Toxins* **2020**, *12*, 602. [CrossRef] [PubMed]
12. Hashemi Yeganeh, H.; Heiat, M.; Kieliszek, M.; Alavian, S.M.; Rezaie, E. DT389-YP7, a Recombinant Immunotoxin against Glypican-3 That Inhibits Hepatocellular Cancer Cells: An In Vitro Study. *Toxins* **2021**, *13*, 749. [CrossRef] [PubMed]
13. Fischer, A.; Wolf, I.; Fuchs, H.; Masilamani, A.P.; Wolf, P. Pseudomonas Exotoxin A Based Toxins Targeting Epidermal Growth Factor Receptor for the Treatment of Prostate Cancer. *Toxins* **2020**, *12*, 753. [CrossRef] [PubMed]

toxins

MDPI

Brief Report

Novel Binding Mechanisms of Fusion Broad Range Anti-Infective Protein Ricin A Chain Mutant-Pokeweed Antiviral Protein 1 (RTAM-PAP1) against SARS-CoV-2 Key Proteins in Silico

Yasser Hassan [1,*], Sherry Ogg [2] and Hui Ge [3]

1 Ophiuchus Medicine Inc., Vancouver, BC V6B 0M3, Canada
2 Biotechnology, Johns Hopkins University, AAP, Baltimore, MD 21218, USA; slojac@gmail.com
3 AscentGene Inc., Gaithersburg, MD 20878, USA; hge@ascentgene.com
* Correspondence: yhassan@ophiuchus.institute

Received: 28 August 2020; Accepted: 14 September 2020; Published: 17 September 2020

Abstract: The deadly pandemic named COVID-19, caused by a new coronavirus (SARS-CoV-2), emerged in 2019 and is still spreading globally at a dangerous pace. As of today, there are no proven vaccines, therapies, or even strategies to fight off this virus. Here, we describe the in silico docking results of a novel broad range anti-infective fusion protein RTAM-PAP1 against the various key proteins of SARS-CoV-2 using the latest protein-ligand docking software. RTAM-PAP1 was compared against the SARS-CoV-2 B38 antibody, ricin A chain, a pokeweed antiviral protein from leaves, and the lectin griffithsin using the special CoDockPP COVID-19 version. These experiments revealed novel binding mechanisms of RTAM-PAP1 with a high affinity to numerous SARS-CoV-2 key proteins. RTAM-PAP1 was further characterized in a preliminary toxicity study in mice and was found to be a potential therapeutic candidate. These findings might lead to the discovery of novel SARS-CoV-2 targets and therapeutic protein structures with outstanding functions.

Keywords: fusion proteins; ricin; pokeweed antiviral protein; COVID-19; SARS-CoV-2; antiviral agent; ribosome-inactivating proteins

Key Contribution: Description of novel binding mechanisms against SARS-COV-2 key proteins resulting from the gain of function of new fusion antiviral protein RTAM-PAP1.

1. Introduction

A new global pandemic disease named COVID-19 has emerged and is still spreading at alarming rates at the time of this report. COVID-19 can cause severe symptoms such as damaging inflammatory response, fever, or severe respiratory illness and lead to death. The causative agent of COVID-19 was found to be a novel coronavirus closely related to the severe acute respiratory syndrome coronavirus (SARS-CoV) based on the latest phylogenetic analysis [1–3]. There are some major essential differences in their genetic makeup that led to their different behaviors. SARS-CoV-2, as it is called now, appears to have high transmissibility from person to person, and antibodies that could inhibit SARS-CoV are not functional on SARS-CoV-2 [2,4,5]. Despite global efforts, we still lack an effective antiviral strategy, drug, or vaccine to fight this virus, with the growing fear that SARS-COV-2 may become another endemic virus in our communities.

To lower the costs and speed up the drug discovery phase, numerous researchers have used in silico tools such as protein–ligand docking software to screen for traditional compounds that could bind to and inhibit the key proteins present in SARS-CoV-2, highlighting their potential antiviral activity [6]. The major targets for these compounds include SARS-CoV-2 key proteins 3-chymotrypsin-like protease

(Mpro), papain-like protease (PLpro), RNA-dependent RNA polymerase (RdRp), small envelope protein (E), membrane protein (M), and spike (S) proteins. The S proteins directly interact with human angiotensin-converting enzyme (ACE2), allowing the virus to enter the cells. The S protein is a class I fusion protein consisting of S1 and S2 domains with the receptor-binding domain (RBD) located on the S1 domain [4]. The RBD is the main target of antibodies and fusion inhibitors in development such as the human convalescent COVID-19 patient-origin B38 antibody (B38) and plant lectin griffithsin (GRFT). Here, we report the in silico potent binding mechanisms against SARS-CoV-2 key proteins of a previously discussed novel broad-spectrum anti-infective fusion protein between a mutant of the ricin A chain and pokeweed antiviral protein isoform 1 (RTAM-PAP1) from seeds of *Ricinus communis* and leaves of *Phytolacca americana*, respectively [7]. RTAM-PAP1 activity was compared with that of the B38, ricin A chain (RTA), pokeweed antiviral protein isolated from leaves (PAP1), and GRFT. Their binding capacities were evaluated against the major key proteins of SARS-CoV-2 using the latest peptide-ligand docking software [8–13].

2. Results

The three-dimensional (3D) structure of RTAM-PAP1 prediction was obtained as previously described [7], and those of RTA, PAP1, B38, and GRFT were retrieved in protein data bank (PDB) format from the Research Collaboratory for Structural Bioinformatics (RCSB) website (https://www.rcsb.org/). A knowledge-based scoring docking prediction was performed for all the compounds against S, S1 RBD, and M using CoDockPP global docking. An additional run was conducted for ACE2 and human SARS-CoV antibody CR3022 against S1 RBD as a reference [5]. The 3D structures of all the key proteins and ACE2 were already available from the software site in this "COVID-19 targets docking only" version. The peptide/antibody–ligand version was used, as small molecules docking software is not suited for these types of compounds. The generated 3D models of B38, ACE2, and CR3022 bound to S1 RBD were comparable to available crystallography of the same complexes in RCSB (access: 7BZ5, 6M0J, and 6W41, respectively) with respective root mean square deviation (RMSD) varying from 0.7 to 4.311 (A), 0.121 to 2.196 (A), and 0.058 to 3.206 (A). However, the greater binding affinity and fusion inhibiting activity of B38 compared to CR3022 for S1 RBD was observed in accordance with published in vitro results [1,3,5]. B38 was found to have a dissociation constant of 70.1 nM with complete inhibition of ACE2 binding to S1 RBD compared to CR3022's dissociation constant of 115 nM with no inhibition of ACE2 binding. The difference in inhibition of ACE2 binding to S1 RBD is due to their binding conformation to S1 RBD. However, ACE2 binding to S1 RBD was found to have the smallest dissociation constant in literature, with a value ranging from 4 to 15 nM. The results for the first and last models (out of the top 10 generated) of each compound in complex with S, S1 RBD, and M are presented in Table 1. B38 has the highest overall binding affinity of the lot with a binding energy ranging from −449 to −300 kcal/mol, as expected. ACE2's binding energy was between −314 to −246 kcal/mol for S1 RBD. RTAM-PAP1 is comparable to B38, with an overall higher binding affinity (lower binding energy) than all of the other compounds tested against the S, S1 RBD, and M key proteins, sometimes higher than B38 with −469 kcal/mol for M, for example. The high binding affinity of RTAM-PAP1 and B38 to S, S1, and M may be explained by the M epitope being very similar in structure to S1 RBD (Figure 1A) [1,3]. RTA binding affinity is similar to RTAM-PAP1 to a certain extent and GRFT and PAP1 are very comparable.

The same higher binding affinity behavior for RTAM-PAP1 was observed with Mpro, PLpro, E, and RdRp when compared to PAP1, GRFT, and RTA (Table 2). All of the tested compounds showed potentially inhibiting binding conformations to the various key proteins based on the 3D structures of the complexes formed (results not shown). These results indicated that the fusion between RTAM and PAP1 allowed RTAM-PAP1 to be more stable across the different possible binding conformations with a higher binding affinity than either of its moieties alone when in complex with SARS-CoV-2 key proteins.

Table 1. The binding energies in kcal/mol for the models generated by CoDockPP for each compound in complex with the outer virus envelope proteins. Top 1 is the model with the lowest binding energy (highest binding affinity) and the top 10 is the 10th model with the lowest binding energy. The lowest energy for the top 1 and top 10 models for each complex is in bold.

Key Proteins	S1 RBD		Spike Trimer		Membrane Protein	
	Top 1	Top 10	Top 1	Top 10	Top 1	Top 10
ACE2	−314	−246				
Compounds						
CR3022	−347	−285				
B38 Antibody	**−367**	**−300**	**−385**	−297	−449	−359
GRFT	−273	−239	−283	−250	−280	−265
RTAM-PAP1	−322	−282	−325	**−298**	**−469**	**−393**
RTA	−322	−278	−313	−275	−387	−348
PAP1	−269	−233	−281	−255	−300	−266

B38 was found to have a 50% inhibition of the cytopathic effect (EC50) against SARS-CoV-2 simultaneous infection in Vero cells in vitro at the concentration of 0.177 µg/mL. It was further demonstrated that B38 was effective in mice post-infection [1]. GRFT was found to have low pre-infection EC50 on different strains of SARS-CoV in cytoprotection (CPE) assays in vitro (0.6–1.2 µg/mL) and effective in mice pre-infection [14]. RTA was shown in the literature to have a high binding affinity to many viral proteins [15,16]. PAP1 has a broad range of antiviral activity against numerous infections both in vitro and in clinical trials [17,18]. An earlier different version of RTAM-PAP1 was shown to have potent broad range antiviral activity at low post-infection EC50 (0.002–12.3 µg/mL) against human immunodeficiency virus-I (HIV), hepatitis B virus (HBV), hepatitis C virus (HCV), Zika virus (Zika), and human coronavirus 229E (HCoV229E) in CPE assays in vitro [7,19]. RTA and PAP1 produce a drastic increase in viral inhibition activity if administered pre-infection both in vitro and in vivo at sub-toxic dosages [20–23], with potent antiviral mechanisms, from viral DNA/RNA depurination, viral proteins synthesis inhibition, viral cell entry inhibition, to apoptosis induction of infected cells via a preferential virus-infected cell entry mechanism [7].

This high affinity of RTAM-PAP1 to many key proteins of SARS-CoV-2 is uncommon. Yet, the most surprising part of the generated models was the discovery of unique binding mechanisms of RTAM-PAP1 with potential inhibiting activity by hindering viral entry and cellular machinery. This discovery might explain the previously observed gain of function of RTAM-PAP1 [7] via the acquired ability to simultaneously bind the target with both moieties with high affinity, i.e., increasing the docking sites from 86 to 102 for single moiety binding and simultaneous binding to S1 RBD, for example. To confirm these findings, RTAM-PAP1 was run against SARS-CoV-2 S1 and M using different docking programs (ZDOCK and HADDOCK2.2) with the known active residues in RCSB. The synergetic binding of RTAM-PAP1 was confirmed, and the generated models for M are shown in Figure 1B–D. Although the model generated by HADDOCK2.2 returned a more important role for PAP1 than RTAM, the simultaneous binding of both moieties can clearly be seen when in complex with M, with an increase in docking sites from 62 for single moiety binding to 96 for simultaneous binding of both moieties (ZDOCK model). This might significantly increase RTAM-PAP1's potential anti-SARS-CoV-2 activity. We concluded from these results and those previously acquired in vitro that the fusion of RTAM and PAP1 via the flexible linker conferred greater structure stability, enhanced activities, new binding sites and mechanisms, and, potentially, novel functions to RTAM-PAP1.

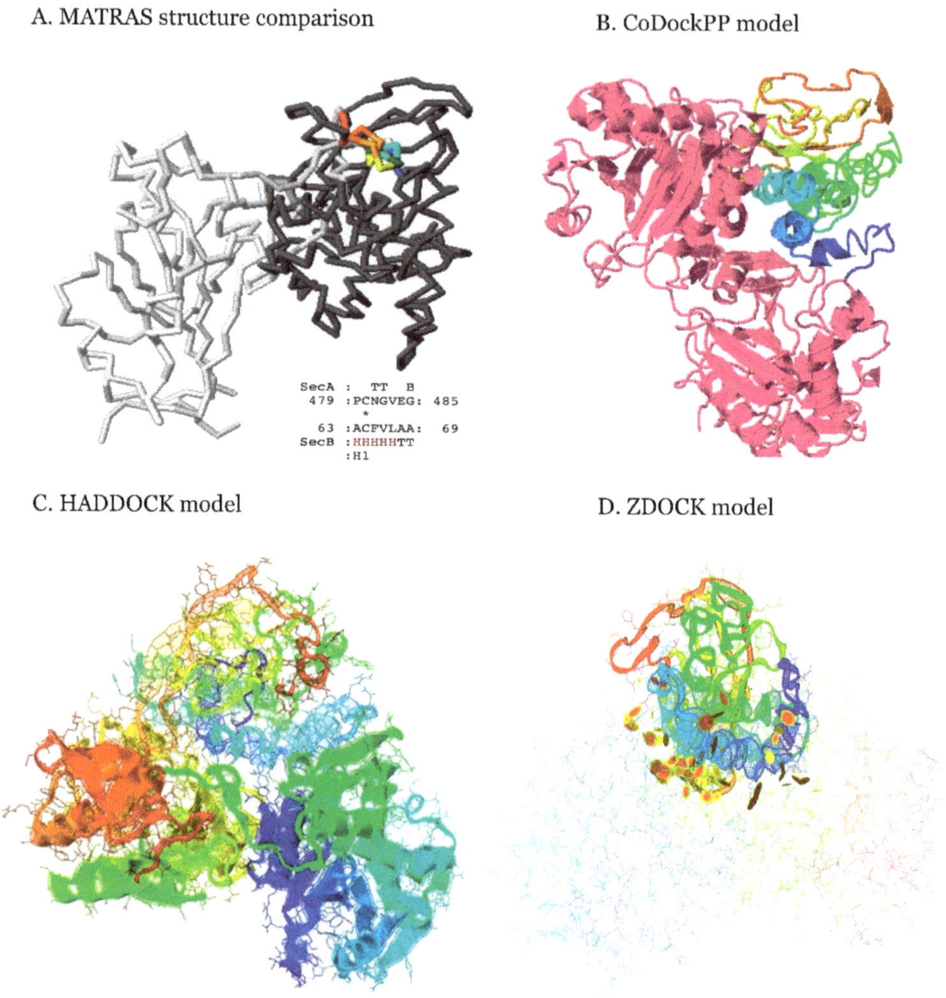

Figure 1. (**A**) Three-dimensional (3D) structure comparison by MATRAS of M protein epitope with S1 protein. M epitope sequence (SecB) is not similar to S1 RBD with only one residue in common (marked with an "*"), yet the structure is similar (depicted in rainbow colors). (**B**) Top model generated by CoDockPP of RTAM-PAP1 (magenta, RTAM being on the upper left side) in complex with M protein (in rainbow colors). (**C**) Top model generated by HADDOCK2.2 with a score of −163.8 (±8.3). PAP1 is on the left side to denote its more important role than in other models and RTAM on the right side (from right to left, N to C terminal in blue to red). M protein is on top and in less solid rainbow colors (N to C terminal in blue to red). (**D**) The top model generated by ZDOCK with RTAM-PAP1 in backbone format (N to C terminal in blue to red). The colored disks depict the binding contact sites. The disks indicate where the van der Waals radii of atoms overlap and the colors how close the contact is: yellow = close, orange = touching, and red = overlapping (models viewed using Jmol).

Table 2. The binding energies in kcal/mol for the models generated by CoDockPP for each compound less the antibody with the viral proteins important for cellular machinery. Top 1 is the model with the lowest binding energy (highest binding affinity) and the top 10 is the 10th model with the lowest binding energy. The lowest energy for the top 1 and top 10 models for each complex is in bold.

Key Proteins	Mpro		Plpro		RdRp		E Protein	
	Top 1	Top 10	Top 1	Top 10	Top 1	Top 10	Top 1	Top 10
Compounds								
GRFT	−228	−198	−234	−209	−267	−248	−258	−242
RTAM-PAP1	**−301**	**−266**	−276	**−259**	**−332**	**−301**	**−363**	**−306**
RTA	−299	−260	**−283**	−254	−304	−277	−314	−281
PAP1	−246	−207	−225	−188	−244	−228	−244	−229

For those reasons, the decision to produce highly purified RTAM-PAP1 protein was taken to conduct a short toxicity study in BALB/c mice to determine the potential maximum tolerated dose.

The protein production went well and followed a scheme previously used [7] with the addition of an endotoxins removal step after purification, as shown in Figure 2A. Highly purified 6-His tag RTAM-PAP1 was obtained (>95% purity), as shown in Figure 2B. The bioactivity of the proteins was confirmed using a cell-free protein synthesis inhibition assay at three different concentrations in duplicate and yielded a half maximal inhibitory concentration (IC50) of 0.06 nM at 60 min incubation time, in line with previous results [7] confirming the time- and concentration-dependent inhibitory activity of RTAM-PAP1 on protein synthesis (data available upon request).

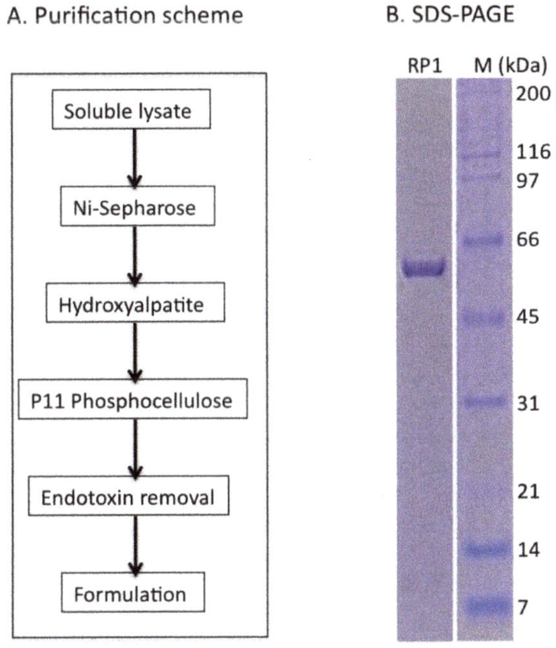

Figure 2. (**A**) Purification scheme and (**B**) purified RTAM-PAP1 protein (RP1). "M" represents protein standards in kilodalton.

The mice were administered the highly purified RTAM-PAP1 with the 6-His tag and tolerated up to 1 mg/kg with no observable adverse effects. Adverse clinical signs were observed (i.e., weight loss, piloerection, etc.) at a single bolus intravenous administration of 3 mg/kg of RTAM-PAP1 with up-regulation of IP-10, KC, and MCP-1 chemokines from 14 cytokines/chemokines assessed (Figure 3). These results are in line with previously described homopolymers of ribosome-inactivating proteins and confirm an in vivo behavior intermediate between native ribosome-inactivating proteins and immunotoxins [24,25].

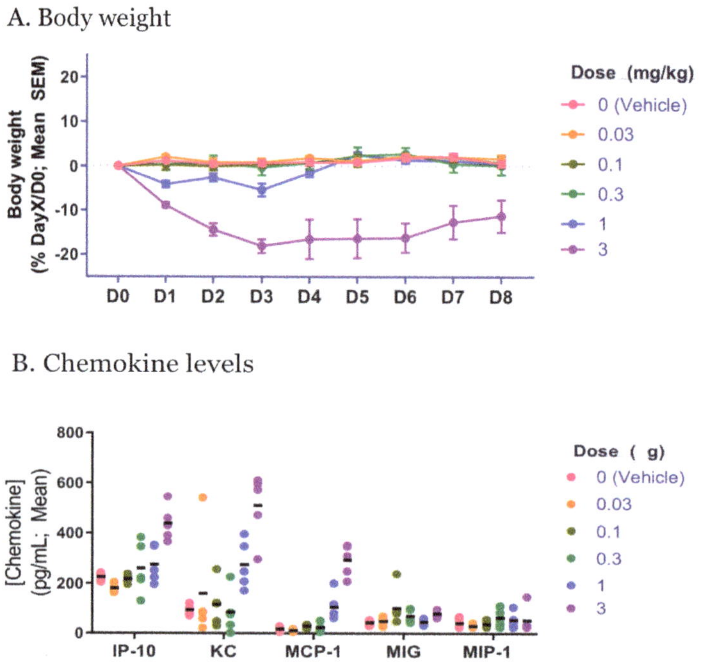

Figure 3. (**A**) Body weight of mice measured daily following administration of various single bolus injection concentrations compared to control. (**B**) Serum chemokine levels measured 3hrs after administration of various single bolus injection concentrations compared to control.

3. Conclusions

In conclusion, given the very high affinity for SARS-CoV-2 key proteins, the previous antiviral results in vitro, the newly discovered mechanisms, the preliminary in vivo profile, potent bioactivities across the assays, and preferential entry into virus-infected cells as opposed to non-infected cells, we opine that this novel chimeric protein composed by two ribosome-inactivating proteins be tested against SARS-CoV-2 in vitro and in vivo. It would be the first therapeutic testing using this particular strategy against COVID-19 and might make a difference at subtoxic dosages as well as open the doors for the discovery of novel SARS-CoV-2 targets, therapeutic protein structures, and foundations for protein engineering. Those types of fusion proteins are able to outperform immunotoxins with lower production costs and less toxicity.

4. Materials and Methods

4.1. Protein Modeling

4.1.1. Generation of 3D Structures

The predicted molecular 3D structure of RTAM-PAP1 was already available from previous work [7] and is available in the supplementary files (PDB file S1). The 3D models for RTA, PAP1, B38, CR3022, and GRFT were retrieved from RCSB (https://www.rcsb.org), in PDB format with the following PDB ID: 4MX5, 1PAG, 7BZ5, 6W41, and 3LL2, respectively). The 3D models for S, Mpro, PLpro, ACE2, RdRp, E, and M were retrieved directly from the CoDockPP site (https://ncov.schanglab.org.cn/). The 3D models for the B38-S1, CR3022-S1 and ACE2-S1 complexes were also retrieved from RCSB, 7BZ5, 6M0J, and 6LZG, respectively, for comparison with CoDockPP outputs.

4.1.2. Structure Modeling

The structure of the bound complexes was generated by CoDockPP using the ambiguous peptide-ligand computations [8–10]. The B38-S1, CR3022-S1, and ACE2-S1 were compared by superimposition on the available crystallography in RCSB using MATRAS pairwise 3D alignment (http://strcomp.protein.osaka-u.ac.jp/matras/matras_pair.html). Additional models of the RTAM-PAP1-S1 and RTAM-PAP1-M complexes were generated using ZDOCK and HADDOCK2.2 [11–13] with the available RCSB active residues as inputs for each protein. The putative active residues for RTAM-PAP1 were previously generated [7] and are available in the supplementary files (Figure S1). All models were viewed using Jmol.

4.2. *Escherichia coli In Vivo Expression System and Rabbit Reticulate Lysate Protein Synthesis Inhibition*

4.2.1. Protein Expression and Purification

RTAM-PAP1 was produced and purified as previously described [7]. The vector pET30a-6H-RPAP1 was generated and validated by DNA sequencing before being transformed into *E. coli* BL21 (DE3) cells (NEB). Expression of the proteins was examined from individual clones and analyzed by either Western blot using a monoclonal antibody specific to ricin A chain (ThermoFisher, RA999, Frederick, MD, USA) or SDS gel stained with Coomassie blue (ThermoFisher, Frederick, MD, USA). Optimal conditions were determined and protein production was induced in the presence of 1 mM isopropyl beta-D-1-thiogalactopyranoside (IPTG) from 1 L culture. The bacteria were then harvested by centrifugation, followed by lysing the cell pellets with 50 mL of lysis buffer (50 mM Tris•Cl, 150 mM NaCl, 0.2% Triton X100, and 0.5 mM ethylenediaminetetraacetic acid (EDTA). After sonication (3×2 min), the soluble lysates were recovered by centrifugation at 35,000 rpm for 40 min. The soluble proteins were then purified by the combination of affinity and conventional chromatographic methods from soluble lysates (please contact the authors for more details). The purification of the native RTAM-PAP1 from soluble lysate was achieved by affinity versus His-tag on the Ni-sepharose column (GE Healthcare). After extensive washing with the lysis buffer, loosely bound proteins were eluted with the lysis buffer containing 40 mM Imidazole (I40). RTAM-PAP1 proteins were eluted with the elution buffer (20 mM Tris•Cl, pH7.9, 100 mM NaCl, 1 mM EDTA, and 300 mM Imidazole). A second purification step using the hydroxyapatite column (GE Healthcare, Piscataway, NJ, USA) was used to further separate RTAM-PAP1 from co-purified host proteins. A third purification step, gel filtration on a fast protein liquid chromatography (FPLC) column of Superose 12 (GE Healthcare, Piscataway, NJ, USA), was necessary to completely remove degraded or/and premature protein products [7]. The resulting mixture was subjected to the endotoxin removal process using a proprietary technology developed by AscentGene until the endotoxin level was less than 10 EU/mL. The final product was formulated in the buffer containing 20 mM HEPES-Na (4-(2-hydroxyethyl)-1-piperazineethanesulfonic acid sodium salt), pH 7.9, 200 mM NaCl, 0.2 mM $CaCl_2$, and 0.5 mM EDTA.

4.2.2. Rabbit Reticulate Lysate Protein Synthesis Inhibition

The inhibitory activities of RTAM-PAP1 were tested by using the Rabbit Reticulate Lysate TnT® Quick Coupled Transcription/Translation System and the Luciferase Assay System (Promega, Madison, WI, USA). Each transcription/translation reaction was performed according to the instructions for use (IFU) in the presence of a T7 Luciferase reporter DNA, and the luciferase expression level was determined with a Wallac Microplate Reader. Transcription/translation were run at three different concentrations to confirm bioactivity [7].

4.3. Preliminary Toxicity Study on Mice

4.3.1. BALB/c Mice

Female BALB/c mice, aged 6–8 weeks (Charles River Laboratories, Saint-Constant, QC, Canada), were used in this study. Female mice were housed in groups of five in individually ventilated cages. The mice were maintained at the National Research Council Canada (NRC) in accordance with the guidelines of the Canadian Council on Animal Care. All procedures performed on animals in this study were in accordance with regulations and guidelines reviewed and approved by the NRC Human Health Therapeutics Ottawa Animal Care Committee.

4.3.2. Animal Procedures

RTAM-PAP1 was administered by intravenous (IV) bolus injection of 0.25 mL into the tail vein in a dose-escalating manner (0.03, 0.1, 0.3, 1, and 3 mg/kg). Control mice received an equivalent volume of vehicle. Dosing was staggered to allow for an initial assessment of tolerability at a particular dose level prior to escalating to a higher dose level. Mice were weighed and evaluated daily for clinical signs for 8 days following administration of RTAM-PAP1. Data were analyzed using GraphPad Prism (GraphPad Software, Inc., San Diego, CA, USA). Statistical significance of the difference between groups was calculated by 1- or 2-factor ANOVA followed by post-hoc analysis. Differences were considered to be not significant at $p > 0.05$.

5. Patent

Hassan, Y. and Ogg, S. WO/2019/204902, The World Intellectual Property Organization (WIPO), 2019.

Supplementary Materials: The following are available online at http://www.mdpi.com/2072-6651/12/9/602/s1, Figure S1: RTAM-PAP1 active sites. PDB file S1: RTAM-PAP1 3D structure.

Author Contributions: Y.H. was responsible for the design, data generation, and for analyses of the in silico experiments. Y.H. was a major contributor to writing the manuscript. S.O. reviewed the in silico experiments and helped in the analysis of the data generated. S.O. revised the entire manuscript critically. H.G. was responsible for protein production, purification, and protein inhibition assays. H.G. was responsible for drafting some of the content of the manuscript and revising critically the entire manuscript. National Research Council of Canada was solely responsible for the preliminary toxicity study on mice. All authors have read and agreed to the published version of the manuscript.

Funding: This work was funded by Ophiuchus Medicine which owns the rights to the patent pending of the fusion protein described in this study. The entire study was done at the request of, by, and for Ophiuchus Medicine.

Acknowledgments: The FP7 WeNMR (project# 261572), H2020 West-Life (project# 675858), and the EOSC-hub (project# 777536) European e-Infrastructure projects are acknowledged for the use of their web portals, which make use of the EGI infrastructure with the dedicated support of CESNET-MCC, INFN-PADOVA, NCG-INGRID-PT, TW-NCHC, SURFsara, and NIKHEF, and the additional support of the national GRID Initiatives of Belgium, France, Italy, Germany, the Netherlands, Poland, Portugal, Spain, U.K., Taiwan, and the U.S. Open Science Grid.

Conflicts of Interest: The authors are either directly or indirectly affiliated to Ophiuchus Medicine. Y.H. and S.O. are officers and shareholders of Ophiuchus Medicine. H.G.'s AscentGene is a subcontractor of Ophiuchus Medicine.

References

1. Wu, Y.; Wang, F.; Shen, C.; Peng, W.; Li, D.; Zhao, C.; Li, Z.; Li, S.; Bi, Y.; Yang, Y.; et al. A noncompeting pair of human neutralizing antibodies block COVID-19 virus binding to its receptor ACE2. *Science* **2020**, *368*, 1274–1278. [CrossRef]
2. Othman, H.; Bouslama, Z.; Brandenburg, J.-T.; Da Rocha, J.; Hamdi, Y.; Ghedira, K.; Srairi-Abid, N.; Hazelhurst, S. Interaction of the spike protein RBD from SARS-CoV-2 with ACE2: Similarity with SARS-CoV, hot-spot analysis and effect of the receptor polymorphism. *Biochem. Biophys. Res. Commun.* **2020**, *527*, 702–708. [CrossRef] [PubMed]
3. Lan, J.; Ge, J.; Yu, J.; Shan, S.; Zhou, H.; Fan, S.; Zhang, Q.; Shi, X.; Wang, Q.; Zhang, L.; et al. Structure of the SARS-CoV-2 spike receptor-binding domain bound to the ACE2 receptor. *Nature* **2020**, *581*, 215–220. [CrossRef] [PubMed]
4. Amawi, H.; Abu Deiab, G.I.; Aljabali, A.A.A.; Dua, K.; Tambuwala, M.M. COVID-19 pandemic: An overview of epidemiology, pathogenesis, diagnostics and potential vaccines and therapeutics. *Ther. Deliv.* **2020**, *11*, 245–268. [CrossRef] [PubMed]
5. Yuan, M.; Wu, N.C.; Zhu, X.; Lee, C.-C.D.; So, R.T.Y.; Lv, H.; Mok, C.K.P.; Wilson, I.A. A highly conserved cryptic epitope in the receptor binding domains of SARS-CoV-2 and SARS-CoV. *Science* **2020**, *368*, 630–633. [CrossRef]
6. Mani, J.S.; Johnson, J.B.; Steel, J.C.; Broszczak, D.A.; Neilsen, P.M.; Walsh, K.B.; Naiker, M. Natural product-derived phytochemicals as potential agents against coronaviruses: A review. *Virus Res.* **2020**, *284*, 197989. [CrossRef]
7. Hassan, Y.; Ogg, S.; Ge, H. Expression of novel fusion antiviral proteins ricin a chain-pokeweed antiviral proteins (RTA-PAPs) in Escherichia coli and their inhibition of protein synthesis and of hepatitis B virus in vitro. *BMC Biotechnol.* **2018**, *18*, 47. [CrossRef]
8. Kong, R.; Yang, G.; Xue, R.; Liu, M.; Wang, F.; Hu, J.; Guo, X.; Chang, S. COVID-19 Docking Server: An interactive server for docking small molecules, peptides and antibodies against potential tar- gets of COVID-19. *arXiv Prepr.* **2020**, arXiv:2003.00163v1.
9. Kong, R.; Wang, F.; Zhang, J.; Wang, F.; Chang, S. CoDockPP: A Multistage Approach for Global and Site-Specific Protein–Protein Docking. *J. Chem. Inf. Model.* **2019**, *59*, 3556–3564. [CrossRef]
10. Trott, O.; Olson, A.J. AutoDock Vina: Improving the speed and accu- racy of docking with a new scoring function, efficient optimization and multithreading. *J. Comput. Chem.* **2010**, *31*, 455–461. [CrossRef]
11. Pierce, B.G.; Wiehe, K.; Hwang, H.; Kim, B.-H.; Vreven, T.; Weng, Z. ZDOCK server: Interactive docking prediction of protein-protein complexes and symmetric multimers. *Bioinformatics* **2014**, *30*, 1771–1773. [CrossRef] [PubMed]
12. van Zundert, G.C.P.; Rodrigues, J.P.G.L.M.; Trellet, M.; Schmitz, C.; Kastritis, P.L.; Karaca, E.; Melquiond, A.S.J.; van Dijk, M.; de Vries, S.J.; Bonvin, A.M.J.J. The HADDOCK2.2 webserver: User-friendly integrative modeling of biomolecular complexes. *J. Mol. Biol.* **2015**, *428*, 720–725. [CrossRef] [PubMed]
13. Wassenaar, T.A.; Van Dijk, M.; Loureiro-Ferreira, N.; Van Der Schot, G.; De Vries, S.J.; Schmitz, C.; Van Der Zwan, J.; Boelens, R.; Giachetti, A.; Ferella, L.; et al. WeNMR: Structural Biology on the Grid. *J. Grid Comput.* **2012**, *10*, 743–767. [CrossRef]
14. O'Keefe, B.R.; Giomarelli, B.; Barnard, D.L.; Shenoy, S.R.; Chan, P.K.; McMahon, J.B.; Palmer, K.E.; Barnett, B.W.; Meyerholz, D.K.; Wohlford-Lenane, C.L.; et al. Broad-Spectrum In Vitro Activity and In Vivo Efficacy of the Antiviral Protein Griffithsin against Emerging Viruses of the Family Coronaviridae. *J. Virol.* **2009**, *84*, 2511–2521. [CrossRef] [PubMed]
15. Olson, M.C.; Ramakrishnan, S.; Anand, R. Ribosomal Inhibitory Proteins from Plants Inhibit HIV-1 Replication in Acutely Infected Peripheral Blood Mononuclear Cells. *AIDS Res. Hum. Retroviruses* **1991**, *7*, 1025–1030. [CrossRef]
16. Ko, S.-M.; Vaidya, B.; Kwon, J.; Lee, H.-M.; Oh, M.-J.; Shin, T.-S.; Cho, S.-Y.; Kim, D. Detection of Hepatitis A Virus in Seeded Oyster Digestive Tissue by Ricin A–Linked Magnetic Separation Combined with Reverse Transcription PCR. *J. Food Prot.* **2015**, *78*, 1046–1051. [CrossRef]
17. Domashevskiy, A.V.; Goss, D.J. Pokeweed Antiviral Protein, a Ribosome Inactivating Protein: Activity, Inhibition and Prospects. *Toxins* **2015**, *7*, 274–298. [CrossRef]

18. Uckun, F.M.; Bellomy, K.; O'Neill, K.; Messinger, Y.; Johnson, T.; Chen, C.L. Toxicity, biological activity, and pharmacokinetics of TXU (anti-CD7)-pokeweed antiviral protein in chimpanzees and adult patients infected with human immunodeficiency virus. *J. Pharmacol. Exp. Ther.* **1999**, *291*, 1301–1307.
19. Hassan, Y.; Ogg, S. *The World Intellectual Property Organization (WIPO)*; The International Bureau of WIPO: Geneva, Switzerland, 2019; Publication number: WO/2019/204902.
20. Teltow, G.J.; Irvin, J.D.; Aron, G.M. Inhibition of herpes simplex virus DNA synthesis by pokeweed antiviral protein. *Antimicrob. Agents Chemother.* **1983**, *23*, 390–396. [CrossRef]
21. Tomlinson, J.A.; Walker, V.M.; Flewett, T.H.; Barclay, G.R. The inhibition of infection by cucumber mosaic virus and influenza virus by extracts from Phytolacca americana. *J Gen. Virol.* **1974**, *22*, 225–232. [CrossRef]
22. Ussery, M.A.; Irvin, J.D.; Hardesty, B. Inhibition of Poliovirus Replication by a Plant Antiviral Peptide. *Ann. N. Y. Acad. Sci.* **1977**, *284*, 431–440. [CrossRef] [PubMed]
23. Ishag, H.Z.; Li, C.; Huang, L.; Sun, M.-X.; Ni, B.; Guo, C.-X.; Mao, X. Inhibition of Japanese encephalitis virus infection in vitro and in vivo by pokeweed antiviral protein. *Virus Res.* **2013**, *171*, 89–96. [CrossRef] [PubMed]
24. Barbieri, L.; Battelli, M.G.; Stirpe, F. Blood clearance and organ distribution and tissue concentration of native, homopolymerized and IgG-conjugated ribosome-inactivating proteins. *Xenobiotica* **1990**, *20*, 1331–1341. [CrossRef] [PubMed]
25. Battelli, M.G.; Barbieri, L.; Stirpe, F. Toxicity of, and histological lesions caused by, ribosome-inactivating proteins, their IgG-conjugates, and their homopolymers. *APMIS* **1990**, *98*, 585–593. [CrossRef]

toxins

MDPI

Review

Immunotoxin Screening System: A Rapid and Direct Approach to Obtain Functional Antibodies with Internalization Capacities

Shusei Hamamichi [1], Takeshi Fukuhara [2,3,4,*] and Nobutaka Hattori [2,3,4]

1. Research Institute for Diseases of Old Age, Juntendo University School of Medicine, Tokyo 113-8421, Japan; s.hamamichi.mo@juntendo.ac.jp
2. Department of Neurology, Juntendo University School of Medicine, Tokyo 113-8421, Japan; nhattori@juntendo.ac.jp
3. Department of Research for Parkinson's Disease, Juntendo University Graduate School of Medicine, Tokyo 113-8421, Japan
4. Neurodegenerative Disorders Collaborative Laboratory, RIKEN Center for Brain Science, Saitama 351-0198, Japan

* Correspondence: noantibody-noscience@umin.ac.jp; Tel.: +81-3-5802-2731; Fax: +81-3-5800-0547

Received: 30 September 2020; Accepted: 14 October 2020; Published: 15 October 2020

Abstract: Toxins, while harmful and potentially lethal, have been engineered to develop potent therapeutics including cytotoxins and immunotoxins (ITs), which are modalities with highly selective targeting capabilities. Currently, three cytotoxins and IT are FDA-approved for treatment of multiple forms of hematological cancer, and additional ITs are tested in the clinical trials or at the preclinical level. For next generation of ITs, as well as antibody-mediated drug delivery systems, specific targeting by monoclonal antibodies is critical to enhance efficacies and reduce side effects, and this methodological field remains open to discover potent therapeutic monoclonal antibodies. Here, we describe our application of engineered toxin termed a cell-based IT screening system. This unique screening strategy offers the following advantages: (1) identification of monoclonal antibodies that recognize cell-surface molecules, (2) selection of the antibodies that are internalized into the cells, (3) selection of the antibodies that induce cytotoxicity since they are linked with toxins, and (4) determination of state-specific activities of the antibodies by differential screening under multiple experimental conditions. Since the functional monoclonal antibodies with internalization capacities have been identified successfully, we have pursued their subsequent modifications beyond antibody drug conjugates, resulting in development of immunoliposomes. Collectively, this screening system by using engineered toxin is a versatile platform, which enables straight-forward and rapid selection for discovery of novel functional antibodies.

Keywords: monoclonal antibody; immunotoxin; antibody drug conjugate; immunoliposome; drug delivery; diphtheria toxin; DT3C

Key Contribution: This review summarizes a current status of immunotoxins including our application of a cell-based screening system to isolate monoclonal antibodies that are suitable for further development as immunotoxins, antibody drug conjugates, and immunoliposomes.

1. Introduction

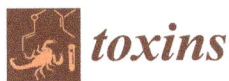

Immunotoxin (IT), a subgroup of immunoconjugates, consists of a target recognition moiety that is linked to bacterial or plant proteineous toxins [1,2]. As an IT, the target recognition moiety is a full-length monoclonal antibody or antibody fragment that specifically binds to an antigen expressed on the surface of target cell, and as a cytotoxin, the component includes a receptor-specific ligand, such as cytokine, chemokine receptor ligand, and growth factor [3,4]. The cytotoxic protein is composed of a toxin derived from bacteria, such as *Pseudomonas aeruginosa* exotoxin A (PE) or diphtheria toxin (DT), as well as from plants including ricin, saporin, gelonin, and bouganin [5–10]. While simple in conceptual design, consisting of two major components, multiple combinations of these two parts allow unlimited prospects to generate potential therapeutic agents with target selectivity. As conceived by Paul Ehrlich with his "magic bullet" concept [11], various types of ITs epitomize potential therapeutic agents with capacities to target disease-relevant antigens.

Current challenges for development of IT as a therapeutic agent include immunogenicity and stability of the fusion protein as well as binding affinity of the target recognition moiety [12]. Here, we overview current toxin-mediated therapeutics, and focus on the target recognition moiety; i.e., monoclonal antibody. Additionally, there are a growing number of highly effective antibody-mediated therapeutics, such as antibody drug conjugates (ADCs). Therefore, we revisit antibody generation technology, beginning from the monumental work on development of the hybridoma technology reported by Köhler and Milstein in 1975 [13], for which they were awarded the Nobel Prize in Physiology and Medicine in 1984. Since then, various advancements for high throughput production of these antibodies have been proposed and reported [14,15]. Here, we compare multiple screening systems to obtain monoclonal antibodies, and describe our unique strategy termed a cell-based IT screening system. The IT screening system, which utilizes distinct features of antibody and engineered toxin, is a rapid, and perhaps more importantly, direct method to identify antibodies that recognize cell surface molecules and are internalized into the cells to induce cytotoxicity. In principle, the selected antibodies through this screening system are suitable for ADCs, immunoliposomes (ILPs) or other drug delivery systems.

2. Current FDA-Approved Toxin-Mediated Therapeutics

Presently, three toxin-mediated therapeutics, such as cytotoxins and IT have been approved by the U.S. Food and Drug Administration (FDA) (Table 1). Denileukin diftitox (Ontak®), administered as an antineoplastic agent for treatment of persistent or recurrent cutaneous T-cell lymphoma, is comprised of a full-length sequence of IL2 protein that is fused to truncated DT (DAB389) [16]. This fusion protein is targeted to the cells expressing interleukin-2 receptor (IL2R), and upon binding, denileukin diftitox is internalized by receptor-mediated endocytosis and proteolytically cleaved to generate a fragment of DT that inhibits protein synthesis by ADP-ribosylation of elongation factor (EF)-2 and induces cytotoxicity [17]. Tagraxofusp (Elzonris®), used for treatment of blastic plasmacytoid dendritic cell neoplasms, is composed of a human IL3 protein and truncated DT [18]. Moxetumomab pasudotox (Lumoxiti®), approved for treatment of relapsed or refractory hairy cell leukemia, consists of a binding fragment (Fv) of anti-cluster of differentiation-22 (CD22) antibody (RFB4) and a 38 kDa portion of PE termed PE38 [19]. Currently, over 20 IT therapeutics are being tested in the clinical trials. As elegantly reviewed by Kim et al. [20], common themes among the FDA-approved toxin-mediated therapeutics include the target recognition moiety that specifically targets hematological cancer cells, and the truncated bacterial toxins that allow reduced levels of immunogenicity and non-specific binding.

In addition to the current FDA-approved therapeutics, multiple toxin-mediated modalities targeting solid tumors are presently in the clinical trials. These modalities include cintredekin besudotox (IL13-PE38QQR) for glioblastoma [28], oportuzumab monatox (VB4-845) for urothelial carcinoma [29], naptumomab estafenatox for renal cell carcinoma [30], and LMB-100 for advanced pancreatic adenocarcinoma [31]. At the preclinical level, ITs have been developed and modified to target activated macrophages [32], murine noradrenergic neurons in the locus ceruleus [33], and human immunodeficiency virus (HIV)-infected cells [34]. While most previous and present ITs and cytotoxins have been designed to target cancer, as long as target selectivity and cytotoxicity are desired, these modalities can conceptually be applied for treatment of various diseases including neuronal diseases.

Table 1. FDA-approved cytotoxins, immunotoxin, and antibody drug conjugates.

Drug Name	Targeting Moiety	Toxin Moiety	Tumor Type	Approval Year	References
		Cytotoxins			
Denileukin diftitox (Ontak®)	IL2	DT (DAB389)	CTCL	1999	[16]
Tagraxofusp-erzs (Elzonris®)	IL3	DT (DAB389)	BPDCN	2018	[18]
		Immunotoxin			
Moxetumomab pasudotox (Lumoxiti®)	Anti-CD22 dsFv	PE (PE38)	HCL	2018	[19]
		Antibody Drug Conjugates			
Gemtuzumab ozogamicin (Mylotarg®)	Humanized anti-CD33 mAb	Ozogamicin	AML	2000-approved 2010-withdrawn 2017-reapproved	[21]
Brentuximab vedotin (Acetris®)	Chimeric anti-CD30 mAb	MMAE	ALCL, HL, PTCL	2011	[22,23]
Trastuzumab emtansine (Kadcyla®)	Humanized anti-HER2 mAb	DM1	HER2$^+$ BC	2013	[24,25]
Inotuzumab ozogamicin (Besponsa®)	Humanized anti-CD22 mAb	Ozogamicin	ALL	2017	[26]
Polatuzumab vedotin (Polivy™)	Humanized anti-CD79B mAb	MMAE	DLBCL	2019	[27]
Enfortumab vedotin (Padcev™)	Human anti-nectin-4 mAb	MMAE	UC	2019	[27]
Trastuzumab deruxtecan (Enhertu®)	Humanized anti-HER2 mAb	Deruxtecan	HER2$^+$ BC	2019	[27]
Sacituzumab govitecan (Trodelvy™)	Humanized anti-Trop-2 mAb	SN-38	Triple-negative BC	2020	[27]

ALCL: anaplastic large cell lymphoma; ALL: acute lymphoblastic leukemia; AML: acute myeloid leukemia; BC: breast cancer; BPDCN: blastic plasmacytoid dendritic cell neoplasm; CTCL: cutaneous T-cell lymphoma; DLBCL: diffuse large B cell lymphoma; DM1: derivative of maytansine 1; DT: diphtheria toxin; HCL: hairy cell leukemia; HER2: human epidermal growth factor receptor 2; HL: Hodgkin lymphoma; mAb: monoclonal antibody; MMAE: monomethyl auristatin E; PE: *Pseudomonas* exotoxin A; PTCL: peripheral T-cell lymphoma; SN-38: active metabolite of irinotecan; UC: urothelial cancer.

For future generation of ITs with enhanced efficacies and reduced adverse events, improved target recognition and reduced immunogenicity are key factors. The latter topic, which focuses on immunogenicities associated with antibodies, and especially bacterial and plant toxins are reviewed elsewhere [35–37] and beyond the scope of this review article. Improvement on target recognition is dependent upon specificity and affinity of monoclonal antibody. Furthermore, given the necessity to deliver the toxin into the cell, internalization of the antibody is pivotal. Regardless of the major advancements, such as humanized ITs [38,39] or bispecific ITs targeting CD19 and CD22 [40,41], quality of the antibody unequivocally remains crucial. Therefore, we must carefully employ an antibody screening strategy that maximizes the attainment of the elite antibody with sufficient internalization capacity suitable for subsequent modification as an IT, ADC or ILP to deliver the payload like toxin. Simultaneously, it is also important to identify disease-specific antigens, especially epitopes.

3. Mode-of-Actions of Therapeutic Antibodies

It is important to emphasize that not all antibody-based therapeutics require internalization capacities since therapeutic efficiencies are dependent on functionalities of the antibodies [42,43]. Monoclonal antibodies, such as rituximab (Rituxan®; a chimeric anti-CD20 monoclonal antibody) and trastuzumab (Herceptin®; a humanized anti-HER2 monoclonal antibody) induce cytotoxicities of target cells via antibody dependent cellular cytotoxicity (ADCC) [44–46]. Through conjunction with radionuclides, such as ^{111}In or ^{90}Y, ibritumomab tiuxetan (Zevalin®; a mouse anti-CD20 monoclonal antibody) is a radioimmunoconjugate with both diagnostic and therapeutic (i.e., theranostic) capacities [47,48]. Bevacizumab [Avastin®; a humanized anti-vascular endothelial growth factor-A (VEGF-A) monoclonal antibody] neutralizes a ligand, which consequently reduces microvascular growth [49,50]. Nivolumab [Opdivo®; a human anti-programmed cell death protein 1 (PD-1) monoclonal antibody] and pembrolizumab (Keytruda®; a humanized anti-PD-1 monoclonal antibody) block PD-1 expressed on the lymphocytes, thus allowing the immune cells to attack cancer cells through modulation of the immune system [51,52]. Currently in Phase 3 clinical trial, photoimmunotherapy is another promising approach wherein a monoclonal antibody is conjugated with IRdye700DX, and localized exposure to near-infrared (NIR) light activates the switch that results in rapid and selective death of targeted cancer cells [53,54]. These are a few among many therapeutic monoclonal antibodies that are not necessary to be internalized, but since our focus includes delivery of the toxin into the cells, internalization capacity cannot be ignored.

4. Internalization Assays to Obtain Monoclonal Antibodies with Internalization Capacities

In case of hybridoma technology, production of monoclonal antibody generally starts with immunization of animals with antigens, followed by isolation of splenocytes. Splenocytes and myeloma cells are fused together to generate hybridomas, and the culture supernatants of these hybridomas need to be screened to identify the candidate antibodies. Subsequent process with limiting dilution enables to establish a hybridoma clone that produces monoclonal antibody. In general, antibody recognizes a structure of corresponding region that consists of approximately 15 amino acids, suggesting that the selection of antibody is affected by the screening methods due to the structural state of target molecule. In other words, the selected antibodies are primarily suitable for the screening methods used. Common assays include immunocytochemistry with fixed cells, enzyme-linked immunosorbent assay (ELISA) with recombinant proteins, and immunoblotting with denatured proteins, but these methods are not always guaranteed to select the potent therapeutic antibodies that recognize the in vivo states of antigens. While these techniques offer notable advantages for selecting antibodies with different characteristics, these procedures are not suitable to determine internalization properties of the antibodies, which are indispensable for most types of drug delivery systems. Therefore, it should be reminded that candidate antibodies have to be screened with consideration for the in vivo structural states of antigenic molecules expressed on the target cells.

As for previous efforts to determine internalization of monoclonal antibody, reported methods are categorized as either direct internalization or indirect internalization assays. Direct internalization assay generally utilizes a purified primary antibody labeled with radioisotope [55] or fluorescence probe [56,57]. These methods possess two obstacles including a necessity to purify primary antibody (hence, supernatants directly obtained from the hybridoma library cannot be used), and a facility that allows the use of radioisotopes or fluorescence scanner. The former issue can be solved by performing indirect internalization assay wherein a purified secondary antibody is labeled, but the latter depends on the facility infrastructure. Additionally, while cellular internalization may sufficiently be measured, subsequent cytotoxicity is not analyzed; hence, internalization and cytotoxicity of IT is more accurate evaluation to assess the potential of the antibody for drug delivery. Additionally, it is feasible to conduct flow cytometry to identify receptor internalization by analyzing the cells with or without PMA stimulation; however, this approach is not suitable for high-throughput screening [58].

Internalization and cytotoxic properties of ITs have been reported through direct labeling with radioisotope [59] or fluorescent dye with functional group [60]. These techniques require purified ITs; therefore, they are inappropriate as a screening procedure to distinguish the hybridomas that secrete desired antibodies from those that do not produce them. More favorable approach is indirect IT assay wherein a toxin-labeled secondary antibody is utilized to identify a monoclonal antibody of interest [61,62]. While successful, since this procedure relies on the toxin-labeled secondary antibody, structural composition is not identical to the final form of IT or ADC where monoclonal (primary) antibody is directly linked to toxins or drugs. Taken together, these issues highlight a major demand to establish an IT screening system with more predictive analysis of the monoclonal antibody.

5. Cell-Based Immunotoxin Screening System

To this end, we previously reported a cell-based IT screening system to facilitate the identification and isolation of monoclonal antibodies with internalization properties [63]. This rapid and direct screening strategy offers the following advantages: (1) identification of monoclonal antibodies that recognize cell-surface molecules, (2) selection of the antibodies that are internalized into the cells, (3) selection of the antibodies that induce cytotoxicity since they are linked with toxins, and (4) determination of state-specific activities of the antibodies by differential screening under multiple experimental conditions. Unlike the procedures described above, our cell-based IT screening system does not require radioisotopes nor fluorescent dyes, and it does not utilize toxin-labeled secondary antibodies. Collectively, our approach provides a platform for direct discovery of potent IT-, ADC- or ILP-compatible antibodies in vitro.

Prior to the IT screening, our approach undergoes three major steps to generate a hybridoma library: (1) immunization, (2) cell-fusion of splenocytes and myeloma cells, and (3) library construction of hybridomas through hypoxanthine-aminopterin-thymidine (HAT) selection. Generation of the hybridoma library is advantageous since hybridoma technology allows continuous growth of hybridomas and production of a large quantity of purified antibodies by conventional method [64]. Additionally, the hybridoma library can be frozen and stored for later studies. To conduct the IT screening, the supernatants from the hybridoma library were pre-incubated with engineered toxin DT3C to form ITs (Figure 1a). DT3C is a recombinant protein that consists of DT without the receptor-binding domain but containing the fragment crystallizable (Fc)-binding domain of *Streptococcus* protein G (3C) [65]. Because of this remarkable feature, DT3C specifically binds to an antibody with affinity. As summarized in Figure 1b, if the IT recognizes a surface molecule expressed on the cell, then the IT is internalized wherein DT3C is cleaved by the cytosolic furin protease, and catalytic domain of DT3C is released into the cytoplasm. The released catalytic domain leads to ADP-ribosylation of EF-2, followed by inhibition of the protein translation machinery and ultimately cytotoxicity.

Utilizing the unique principle of our IT assay system, we performed primary screening to identify antibody-secreting hybridomas that were capable of inducing DT3C-dependent cytotoxicity (Figure 1c). Induction of cytotoxicity was assessed by WST-1 assay to quantitatively evaluate cell viability. We established 90G4 clone that produced functional monoclonal antibody with capacity for DT3C-dependent cytotoxicity [63]. Subsequently, 90G4, a rat anti-mouse CD321/F11 receptor antibody was further characterized by flow cytometry, immunocytochemistry, immunoprecipitation, immunoblotting, and mass spectrometry, demonstrating differential expression patterns of CD321 under normoxic vs. hypoxic conditions. This study revealed new roles of endothelial CD321 that was internalized upon the hypoxic signal. While we utilized the hybridoma technology to generate monoclonal antibodies, it is noteworthy that, in principle, our cell-based IT screening system is applicable to the screening of the antibodies obtained from antibody phage display [66–68] and single B cell antibody technologies [69,70].

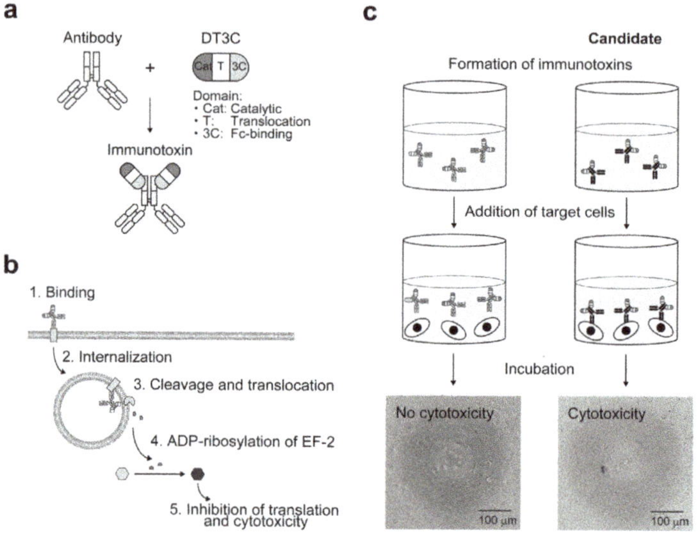

Figure 1. Mechanism of antibody: DT3C IT. (**a**) Formation of DT3C-mediated IT. DT3C consists of catalytic (Cat), translocation (T), and Fc-binding (3C) domains. The Fc-binding domain of DT3C specifically binds to an antibody. (**b**) Mechanism of IT-induced cytotoxicity. IT initially binds to an antigen expressed on the cell surface, and internalized into the cell where translocated terminus of DT3C is cleaved by the cellular furin protease, and catalytic domain of DT3C is released into the cytoplasm. Consequently, the catalytic domain ADP-ribosylates EF-2 and inhibits the protein translation machinery. (**c**) Cell-based IT screening system. Inside a well of the cell culture plate, antibodies secreted into the supernatant of the hybridoma library are pretreated with DT3C to form ITs. Subsequently, target cells are transferred into the well, and incubated. If the IT is bound to the target cells and internalized, then this leads to inhibition of protein translation machinery and ultimately cytotoxicity.

6. Application of Functional Monoclonal Antibodies as Antibody Drug Conjugates

ADCs have gained significant attention as highly potent therapeutic agents because of their pharmacological characteristics including target specificity, target-binding affinity, good retention, and low immunogenicity that altogether contribute to targeted drug delivery and decreased side effects [71–74]. Accordingly, FDA-approved ADCs include gemtuzumab ozogamicin (Mylotarg®; a humanized anti-CD33 monoclonal antibody conjugated to ozogamicin) for CD33-positive acute myeloid leukemia [21,75]; brentuximab vedotin [Acetris®; a chimeric anti-CD30 monoclonal antibody conjugated to monomethyl auristatin E (MMAE)] for relapsed Hodgkin lymphoma, systemic anaplastic large cell lymphoma, and other CD30-expressing peripheral T-cell lymphomas [22,23]; trastuzumab emtansine (Kadcyla®; a humanized anti-HER2 monoclonal antibody conjugated to DM1) for HER2-positive breast cancer [24,25]; and inotuzumab ozogamicin (Besponsa®; a humanized anti-CD22 monoclonal antibody conjugated to ozogamicin) for acute lymphoblastic leukemia [26] (Table 1). Recently, four additional ADCs have been FDA-approved; polatuzumab vedotin (Polivy™; a humanized anti-CD79B monoclonal antibody conjugated to MMAE) for diffuse large B cell lymphoma, enfortumab vedotin (Padcev™; a human anti-nectin-4 monoclonal antibody conjugated to MMAE) for urothelial cancer, trastuzumab deruxtecan (Enhertu®; a humanized anti-HER2 monoclonal antibody conjugated to deruxtecan) for unresectable or metastatic HER2-positive breast cancer, and sacituzumab govitecan (Trodelvy™; a humanized anti-Trop-2 monoclonal antibody conjugated to SN-38) for metastatic triple-negative breast cancer [27].

Typically, ADC consists of a monoclonal antibody that is linked to cytotoxic payloads by non-cleavable or cleavable linker [71–74]. Similar to IT, quality of the monoclonal antibody is crucial because therapeutic property of ADC is partially related to the characteristics of its antigen. Specifically, not only are differential surface expression levels of antigens between the target and non-target cells essential, the antigens are preferred to possess internalization properties because it will facilitate the ADC to be transported into the cells and enhance its efficacy. The notion was also illustrated for generation of ADC by using a human single chain variable fragment (scFv)-Fc antibody against CD239/basal cell adhesion molecule for treatment of breast cancer [76]. The scFV-Fc antibody termed C7-Fc, originally identified from screening the scFv phage libraries [77], was bound to DT3C to characterized its internalization property, and selectively target and kill SKBR3 breast cancer cells. This work also provides evidence supporting the application of our cell-based IT screening system to characterize the candidates identified from the phage display libraries.

From the IT screening method, a mouse anti-human CD71/transferrin receptor antibody termed 6E1 antibody was identified and isolated [65]. To assess its cytotoxic potential, purified 6E1 antibody was pretreated with DT3C and administered to A172, SH-SY5Y, and H4 cells. As an IT, 6E1:DT3C demonstrated strong cytotoxic activities wherein logEC50s (ng/mL) were 4.59 (A172), 2.27 (SH-SY5Y), and 6.87 (H4) (Figure 2). To generate its ADC form, antibody binding peptide termed Z33 was elegantly conjugated with anti-cancer agent plinabulin, and Z33-conjugated plinabulin was then used to non-covalently bind to 6E1 antibody [78]. As expected, this ADC demonstrated enhanced cytotoxicity against CD71-positive melanoma A375 cells. In addition to the 6E1 antibody, mouse anti-human Mucin 13 (MUC13) antibody termed TCC56 was identified from the IT screening method and shown to induce cell death in TCC-PAN2 cells expressing MUC13 [79].

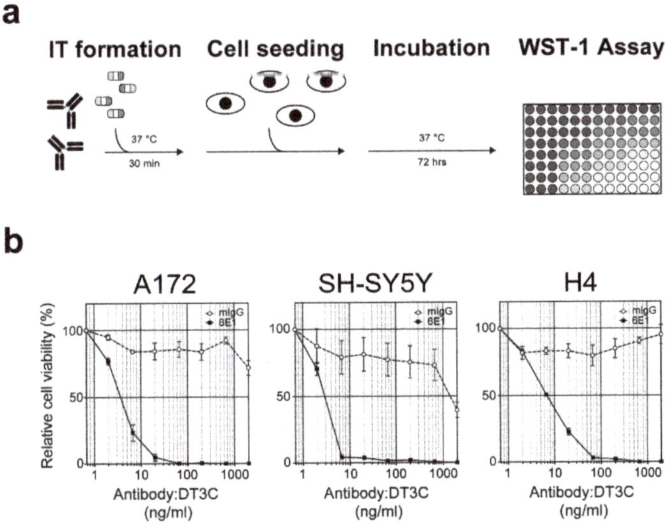

Figure 2. Cytotoxic activity of 6E1:DT3C IT. (**a**) Schematic diagram of IT assay. Purified 6E1 or control mouse IgG (mIgG) antibodies were pre-incubated with DT3C at 37 °C for 30 min to form ITs. After the IT formation, the indicated cells were seeded with various concentrations of ITs (n = 3 per treatment) and incubated at 37 °C for 3 days. Cell viability was measured by using WST-1 reagent. (**b**) Relative cell viability of A172, SH-SY5Y, and H4 cell lines after 6E1:DT3C treatment. The 6E1:DT3C IT induced cytotoxicity in all three cells lines tested whereby the logEC50s (ng/mL) were 4.59 (A172), 2.27 (SH-SY5Y), and 6.87 (H4). Assuming that 2 DT3Cs (75 kDa each) bind to one antibody, antibody:DT3C at 2000 ng/mL corresponds to 13 nM. Representative results of triplicate independent experiments. Data represent AVG ± SD.

7. Challenges for Next Generation of Antibody Drug Conjugates

Optimization of monoclonal antibody, linker, and cytotoxic payload, as well as increased retention and enhanced penetration to the target cells are key factors associated with improved next generation of ADCs that will enhance efficacies and reduce side effects [71–74]. Moreover, one of the critical features to consider for development of ADCs as drug delivery modalities is drug-to-antibody ratio (DAR). For instance, high DAR affects antibody structure and stability, and low DAR can decrease efficacy; therefore, in most cases, their DAR values are restricted to the manageable ranges [80,81]. Recently, Ogitani et al. reported that a HER2-targeting ADC termed DS-8201a was successfully conjugated with 8 molecules of novel topoisomerase I inhibitors per antibody, and that this ADC exhibited potent anti-tumor activities in a wide range of HER2-positive animal models with favorable pharmacokinetics and safety profiles [82]. To maximize drug load and minimize structural changes and instability of the monoclonal antibody, one avenue to explore is generation of ILP.

8. Application of Functional Monoclonal Antibodies as Immunoliposomes

There are numerous advantages to liposomes, such as biocompatibility, biodegradability, low toxicity, and their capacities to encapsulate both hydrophilic and hydrophobic drugs [83,84]. Conventional liposomes are phospholipid bilayers that are composed of certain molar ratios of phospholipids and cholesterols with drugs entrapped inside. To prolong blood circulation time and reduce uptake by the cells of the reticuloendothelial system, polyethylene glycol (PEG) was added to the surface of the liposomes termed "stealth" liposomes. Consequently, multiple formulations of conventional and PEGylated liposomes have been FDA-approved including Doxil®, DaunoXome®, Depocyt®, Marqibo®, Onivyde® and Vyxeos® for various forms of cancer, as well as Amphotec® and Ambisome® for fungal infections [85–88]. Potential candidates for liposomal encapsulation include clinically approved or presently developed therapeutic agents for treatment of cancer, neurodegenerative diseases, cardiovascular diseases, inflammation, and infections [89,90]. Moreover, combined with imaging modalities, such as magnetic resonance imaging (MRI), ultrasound, single-photon emission computed tomography (SPECT), and positron emission tomography (PET), MRI- or ultrasound-contrast agents, as well as radionuclides can be encapsulated into the liposomes for diagnostic, therapeutic, and potentially theranostic application [91–94].

To introduce novel functionalities to the liposomes, monoclonal antibodies or their fragments, such as fragment antigen-binding (Fab) or scFv, are conjugated to the liposomal surface to generate ILPs [95,96]. Given the clinical success of Doxil® (PEGylated liposome encapsulating anti-cancer agent doxorubicin) [97], next endeavor was active targeting to attain improved drug delivery and therapeutic efficacy. Park et al. generated anti-HER2 ILP that encapsulated doxorubicin, and reported identical prolonged blood circulation compared with control PEGylated liposome without antibody conjugation, as well as enhanced therapeutic outcomes in four different HER2-overexpressing tumor xenograft models [98]. Furthermore, anti-HER2 ILP that encapsulated paclitaxel and rapamycin also demonstrated controlled tumor growth in a mouse orthotopic HER2-positive SKBR3 xenograft model [99]. Conversely, a lack of increased anti-tumor activity after ILP administration has also been reported [100]. Considering the heterogenous and complex nature of cancer, drug delivery, tumor accumulation of the ILPs, internalization of the encapsulated drugs, and multiple additional factors combined contribute to therapeutic efficiencies [101–104]. Collectively, ILP is a bifunctional modality that possesses the qualities of antibody and liposome with unequivocal potential for targeting specificity and delivery of immensely encapsulated drugs.

In addition to development of cancer therapeutics, at the preclinical level, another intriguing concept is delivery of drugs across the blood brain barrier (BBB) into the brain by using ILPs. The BBB, where cell membrane proteins involved in receptor-mediated transcytosis, such as transferrin receptor and insulin receptor are expressed, is a selective barrier between systemic blood circulation and brain parenchyma [105–108]. Recently, Johnsen et al. reported that intravenous injection of OX26 (a mouse anti-rat CD71/transferrin receptor monoclonal antibody)-conjugated and oxaliplatin-encapsulated liposome resulted in higher concentration of platinum in the rat brain parenchyma compared to the control ILP [109]. We have also tested the application of functional monoclonal antibody as an ILP whereby purified 6E1 antibody was conjugated with $DiOC_{18}(3)$-encapsulated liposome, and the resulting ILP was applied to A172 cells. We observed 5.01-fold increase of cellular uptake at 60 hrs after treatment of 30 μM 6E1-conjugated liposome when compared with the control ILP (Figure 3). Alternatively, HIRMAb (a rabbit anti-insulin receptor monoclonal antibody)-conjugated liposome encapsulating plasmid encoding β-galactosidase was generated, and intravenously injected to Rhesus monkey to demonstrate global expression of β-galactosidase in the primate brain [110,111]. Given the nearly impermeable nature of the BBB, successful drug delivery to the brain through receptor-mediated transcytosis and subsequently to the neurons through endocytosis promises to unlock innovative advancements toward ameliorating neurodegenerative diseases.

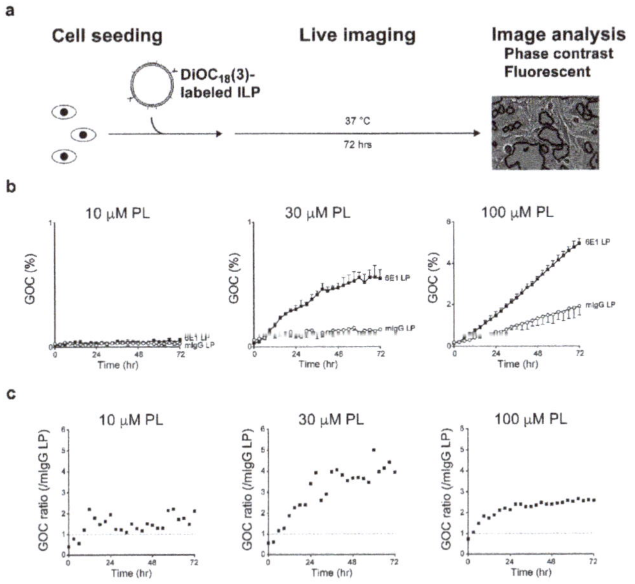

Figure 3. Cellular uptake of 6E1-conjugated liposome. (**a**) Schematic diagram of cellular uptake procedure. Liposomes were initially generated through dissolution of lipids in ethanol, injection of the ethanol solution into aqueous buffer, and extrusion through polycarbonate membranes. Following the extrusion, the liposomes were conjugated with 6E1 or control mouse IgG (mIgG) antibodies, and fluorescently labeled with $DiOC_{18}(3)$. A172 cells and ILPs were simultaneously transferred to a 96-well plate. The cells were treated with the indicated phospholipid (PL) concentrations of ILPs ($n = 3$ per treatment), and incubated at 37 °C for 3 days. Phase contrast and fluorescent images were acquired by using IncuCyte ZOOM (Essen BioScience, Inc.; Ann Arbor, MI, USA). Green fluorescent areas were determined as percentage of green object confluency (GOC). (**b**) Enhanced uptake of 6E1-conjugated liposome. At 100 μM, 6E1-conjugated liposome was significantly taken up by the cells, and mIgG-conjugated liposome also demonstrated gradual increase of cellular uptake. At 30 μM, 6E1-conjugated liposome demonstrated recurrent increased cellular uptake while the control remained relatively low. At 10 μM, cellular uptake of both ILPs remained constantly similar. Representative results of triplicate independent experiments. Data represent AVG ± SD. (**c**) Ratio of GOC between 6E1-conjugated and control mIgG-conjugated liposomes. If there was no difference in cellular uptake between these ILPs, then the ratio would remain at 1 as indicated by dotted lines. The most enhanced difference was observed at 30 μM liposomal concentration wherein 6E1-conjugated liposome exhibited 5.01-fold (60 hrs) increase of the cellular uptake when compared to the control. Representative results of triplicate independent experiments.

9. Future Directions

A common theme among optimized ITs, ADCs, and ILPs is the quality of monoclonal antibody, and there will always be a need to generate the antibody that is translatable to the clinic. As described in this review, a proper screening strategy to pinpoint the antibody of interest is critical. Our cell-based IT screening system closely resembles the structural compositions of ITs and ADCs. As we expand our knowledge on critical features associated with methodological efficiencies and therapeutic efficacies, we can design and modify the screening strategies accordingly including inclusions of antibody phage display and single B cell antibody technologies. These advancements allow us to evaluate multiple feasibilities to maximize the potentials of the antibodies including, but not limited to, ITs, ADCs, and ILPs.

10. Conclusions

In this review, we described a current status of ITs, including our application of ITs as a cell-based IT screening system to obtain monoclonal antibodies that are suitable for further development. Our screening system, which exploits unique characteristics of antibody and engineered toxin DT3C, is a strategy to identify and isolate hybridomas that produce monoclonal antibodies that bind to cell surface molecules and are internalized into the cells to induce cytotoxicity. This system, both rapid and direct, is a platform for discovery of novel IT-, ADC-, and ILP-compatible monoclonal antibodies in vitro.

Author Contributions: Conceptualization: S.H. and T.F.; Writing: S.H. and T.F.; Review and editing: S.H., T.F. and N.H. All authors have read and agreed to the published version of the manuscript.

Funding: This study was partly supported by KAKENHI, a Grant-in-Aid for Scientific Research C (S.H.: 18K07657, T.F.: 16K07184, 19K07831). This research was supported by AMED under Grant Number JP19cm0106231s0102 and JP19dm0107156h0001 (T.F.).

Acknowledgments: We acknowledge the cooperative spirit of all members of the laboratory, and secretaries at the Department of Neurology, Juntendo University.

Conflicts of Interest: The authors declare no conflict of interest.

References

1. Pastan, I.; Hassan, R.; Fitzgerald, D.J.; Kreitman, R.J. Immunotoxin therapy of cancer. *Nat. Rev. Cancer* **2006**, *6*, 559–565. [CrossRef] [PubMed]
2. Allahyari, H.; Heidari, S.; Ghamgosha, M.; Saffarian, P.; Amani, J. Immunotoxin: A new tool for cancer therapy. *Tumor Biol.* **2017**, *39*. [CrossRef] [PubMed]
3. Pastan, I.; Hassan, R.; FitzGerald, D.J.; Kreitman, R.J. Immunotoxin treatment of cancer. *Annu. Rev. Med.* **2007**, *58*, 221–237. [CrossRef] [PubMed]
4. Spiess, K.; Jeppesen, M.G.; Malmgaard-Clausen, M.; Krzywkowski, K.; Kledal, T.N.; Rosenkilde, M.M. Novel chemokine-based immunotoxins for potent and selective targeting of cytomegalovirus infected cells. *J. Immunol. Res.* **2017**, *2017*. [CrossRef] [PubMed]
5. Antignani, A.; Fitzgerald, D. Immunotoxins: The role of the toxin. *Toxins* **2013**, *5*, 1486–1502. [CrossRef] [PubMed]
6. Weidle, U.H.; Tiefenthaler, G.; Schiller, C.; Weiss, E.H.; Georges, G.; Brinkmann, U. Prospects of bacterial and plant protein-based immunotoxins for treatment of cancer. *Cancer Genom. Proteom.* **2014**, *11*, 25–38.
7. Akbari, B.; Farajnia, S.; Khosroshahi, S.A.; Safari, F.; Yousefi, M.; Dariushnejad, H.; Rahbarnia, L. Immunotoxins in cancer therapy: Review and update. *Int. Rev. Immunol.* **2017**, *36*, 207–219. [CrossRef]
8. Bortolotti, M.; Bolognesi, A.; Polito, L. Bouganin, an attractive weapon for immunotoxins. *Toxins* **2018**, *10*, 323. [CrossRef]
9. Polito, L.; Bortolotti, M.; Battelli, M.G.; Calafato, G.; Bolognesi, A. Ricin: An ancient story for a timeless plant toxin. *Toxins* **2019**, *11*, 324. [CrossRef]
10. Lu, J.Q.; Zhu, Z.N.; Zheng, Y.T.; Shaw, P.C. Engineering of ribosome-inactivating proteins for improving pharmacological properties. *Toxins* **2020**, *12*, 167. [CrossRef]

11. Strebhardt, K.; Ullrich, A. Paul Ehrlich's magic bullet concept: 100 years of progress. *Nat. Rev. Cancer* **2008**, *8*, 473–480. [CrossRef]
12. Shan, L.; Liu, Y.; Wang, P. Recombinant immunotoxin therapy of solid tumors: Challenges and strategies. *J. Basic Clin. Med.* **2013**, *2*, 1–6.
13. Köhler, G.; Milstein, C. Continuous cultures of fused cells secreting antibody of predefined specificity. *Nature* **1975**, *256*, 495–497. [CrossRef] [PubMed]
14. Chiarella, P.; Fazio, V.M. Mouse monoclonal antibodies in biological research: Strategies for high-throughput production. *Biotechnol. Lett.* **2008**, *30*, 1303–1310. [CrossRef] [PubMed]
15. Layton, D.; Laverty, C.; Nice, E.C. Design and operation of an automated high-throughput monoclonal antibody facility. *Biophys. Rev.* **2013**, *5*, 47–55. [CrossRef]
16. Lansigan, F.; Stearns, D.M.; Foss, F. Role of denileukin diftitox in the treatment of persistent or recurrent cutaneous T-cell lymphoma. *Cancer Manag. Res.* **2010**, *2*, 53–59. [CrossRef]
17. Bacha, P.; Williams, D.P.; Waters, C.; Williams, J.M.; Murphy, J.R.; Strom, T.B. Interleukin 2 receptor-targeted cytotoxicity. Interleukin 2 receptor-mediated action of a diphtheria toxin-related interleukin 2 fusion protein. *J. Exp. Med.* **1988**, *167*, 612–622. [CrossRef]
18. Jen, E.Y.; Gao, X.; Li, L.; Zhuang, L.; Simpson, N.E.; Aryal, B.; Wang, R.; Przepiorka, D.; Shen, Y.L.; Leong, R.; et al. FDA approval summary: Tagraxofusp-erzs for treatment of blastic plasmacytoid dendritic cell neoplasm. *Clin. Cancer Res.* **2020**, *26*, 532–536. [CrossRef]
19. Lin, A.Y.; Dinner, S.N. Moxetumomab pasudotox for hairy cell leukemia: Preclinical development to FDA approval. *Blood Adv.* **2019**, *3*, 2905–2910. [CrossRef]
20. Kim, J.S.; Jun, S.Y.; Kim, Y.S. Critical issues in the development of immunotoxins for anticancer therapy. *J. Pharm. Sci.* **2020**, *109*, 104–115. [CrossRef]
21. Jen, E.Y.; Ko, C.W.; Lee, J.E.; Del Valle, P.L.; Aydanian, A.; Jewell, C.; Norsworthy, K.J.; Przepiorka, D.; Nie, L.; Liu, J.; et al. FDA approval: Gemtuzumab ozogamicin for the treatment of adults with newly diagnosed CD33-positive acute myeloid leukemia. *Clin. Cancer Res.* **2018**, *24*, 3242–3246. [CrossRef] [PubMed]
22. Deng, C.; Pan, B.; O'Connor, O.A. Brentuximab vedotin. *Clin. Cancer Res.* **2013**, *19*, 22–27. [CrossRef]
23. Richardson, N.C.; Kasamon, Y.L.; Chen, H.; de Claro, R.A.; Ye, J.; Blumenthal, G.M.; Farrell, A.T.; Pazdur, R. FDA approval summary: Brentuximab vedotin in first-line treatment of peripheral T-cell lymphoma. *Oncologist* **2019**, *24*, e180–e187. [CrossRef] [PubMed]
24. Boyraz, B.; Sendur, M.A.N.; Aksoy, S.; Babacan, T.; Roach, E.C.; Kizilarslanoglu, M.C.; Petekkaya, I.; Altundag, K. Trastuzumab emtansine (T-DM1) for HER2-positive breast cancer. *Curr. Med. Res. Opin.* **2013**, *29*, 405–414. [CrossRef]
25. Wedam, S.; Fashoyin-Aje, L.; Gao, X.; Bloomquist, E.; Tang, S.; Sridhara, R.; Goldberg, K.B.; King-Kallimanis, B.L.; Theoret, M.R.; Ibrahim, A.; et al. FDA approval summary: Ado-trastuzumab emtansine for the adjuvant treatment of HER2-positive early breast cancer. *Clin. Cancer Res.* **2020**. [CrossRef]
26. Yurkiewicz, I.R.; Muffly, L.; Liedtke, M. Inotuzumab ozogamicin: A CD22 mAb-drug conjugate for adult relapsed or refractory B-cell precursor acute lymphoblastic leukemia. *Drug Des. Devel. Ther.* **2018**, *12*, 2293–2300. [CrossRef] [PubMed]
27. Mullard, A. 2019 FDA drug approvals. *Nat. Rev. Drug Discov.* **2019**, *18*, 85–89. [CrossRef]
28. Kunwar, S.; Chang, S.; Westphal, M.; Vogelbaum, M.; Sampson, J.; Barnett, G.; Shaffrey, M.; Ram, Z.; Piepmeier, J.; Prados, M.; et al. Phase III randomized trial of CED of IL13-PE38QQR vs. gliadel wafers for recurrent glioblastoma. *Neuro Oncol.* **2010**, *12*, 871–881. [CrossRef] [PubMed]
29. Kowalski, M.; Guindon, J.; Brazas, L.; Moore, C.; Entwistle, J.; Cizeau, J.; Jewett, M.A.S.; MacDonald, G.C. A phase II study of oportuzumab monatox: An immunotoxin therapy for patients with noninvasive urothelial carcinoma in situ previously treated with Bacillus Calmette-Guérin. *J. Urol.* **2012**, *188*, 1712–1718. [CrossRef]
30. Hawkins, R.E.; Gore, M.; Shparyk, Y.; Bondar, V.; Gladkov, O.; Ganev, T.; Harza, M.; Polenkov, S.; Bondarenko, I.; Karlov, P.; et al. A randomized phase II/III study of naptumomab estafenatox + IFNα versus IFNα in renal cell carcinoma: Final analysis with baseline biomarker subgroup and trend analysis. *Clin. Cancer Res.* **2016**, *22*, 3172–3181. [CrossRef]
31. Alewine, C.; Ahmad, M.; Peer, C.J.; Hu, Z.I.; Lee, M.J.; Yuno, A.; Kindrick, J.D.; Thomas, A.; Steinberg, S.M.; Trepel, J.B.; et al. Phase I/II study of the mesothelin-targeted immunotoxin LMB-100 with nab-paclitaxel for patients with advanced pancreatic adenocarcinoma. *Clin. Cancer Res.* **2020**, *26*, 828–836. [CrossRef]

32. Thepen, T.; van Vuuren, A.J.; Kiekens, R.C.; Damen, C.A.; Vooijs, W.C.; van De Winkel, J.G. Resolution of cutaneous inflammation after local elimination of macrophages. *Nat. Biotechnol.* **2000**, *18*, 48–51. [CrossRef]
33. Itoi, K.; Sugimoto, N.; Suzuki, S.; Sawada, K.; Das, G.; Uchida, K.; Fuse, T.; Ohara, S.; Kobayashi, K. Targeting of locus ceruleus noradrenergic neurons expressing human interleukin-2 receptor α-subunit in transgenic mice by a recombinant immunotoxin anti-Tac(Fv)-PE38: A study for exploring noradrenergic influence upon anxiety-like and depression-like behaviors. *J. Neurosci.* **2011**, *31*, 6132–6139. [PubMed]
34. Sadraeian, M.; Guimarães, F.E.G.; Araújo, A.P.U.; Worthylake, D.K.; LeCour, L.J.; Pincus, S.H. Selective cytotoxicity of a novel immunotoxin based on pulchellin A chain for cells expressing HIV envelope. *Sci. Rep.* **2017**, *7*. [CrossRef]
35. Flavell, D.J. Countering immunotoxin immunogenicity. *Br. J. Cancer* **2016**, *114*, 1177–1179. [CrossRef]
36. Grinberg, Y.; Benhar, I. Addressing the immunogenicity of the cargo and of the targeting antibodies with a focus on deimmunized bacterial toxins and on antibody-targeted human effector proteins. *Biomedicines* **2017**, *5*, 28. [CrossRef] [PubMed]
37. Mazor, R.; King, E.M.; Pastan, I. Strategies to reduce the immunogenicity of recombinant immunotoxins. *Am. J. Pathol.* **2018**, *188*, 1736–1743. [CrossRef] [PubMed]
38. Zhang, Y.F.; Ho, M. Humanization of high-affinity antibodies targeting glypican-3 in hepatocellular carcinoma. *Sci. Rep.* **2016**, *6*. [CrossRef]
39. Yu, Y.; Li, J.; Zhu, X.; Tang, X.; Bao, Y.; Sun, X.; Huang, Y.; Tian, F.; Liu, X.; Yang, L. Humanized CD7 nanobody-based immunotoxins exhibit promising anti-T-cell acute lymphoblastic leukemia potential. *Int. J. Nanomed.* **2017**, *12*, 1969–1983. [CrossRef]
40. Bachanova, V.; Frankel, A.E.; Cao, Q.; Lewis, D.; Grzywacz, B.; Verneris, M.R.; Ustun, C.; Lazaryan, A.; McClune, B.; Warlick, E.D.; et al. Phase I study of a bispecific ligand-directed toxin targeting CD22 and CD19 (DT2219) for refractory B-cell malignancies. *Clin. Cancer Res.* **2015**, *21*, 1267–1272. [CrossRef]
41. Schmohl, J.U.; Todhunter, D.; Taras, E.; Bachanova, V.; Vallera, D.A. Development of a deimmunized bispecific immunotoxin dDT2219 against B-Cell malignancies. *Toxins* **2018**, *10*, 32. [CrossRef] [PubMed]
42. Weiner, G.J. Building better monoclonal antibody-based therapeutics. *Nat. Rev. Cancer* **2015**, *15*, 361–370. [CrossRef] [PubMed]
43. Carter, P.J.; Lazar, G.A. Next generation antibody drugs: Pursuit of the 'high-hanging fruit'. *Nat. Rev. Drug Discov.* **2018**, *17*, 197–223. [CrossRef] [PubMed]
44. Clynes, R.A.; Towers, T.L.; Presta, L.G.; Ravetch, J.V. Inhibitory Fc receptors modulate in vivo cytotoxicity against tumor targets. *Nat. Med.* **2000**, *6*, 443–446. [CrossRef] [PubMed]
45. Nahta, R.; Esteva, F.J. Trastuzumab: Triumphs and tribulations. *Oncogene* **2007**, *26*, 3637–3643. [CrossRef]
46. Weiner, G.J. Rituximab: Mechanism of action. *Semin. Hematol.* **2010**, *47*, 115–123. [CrossRef]
47. Emmanouilides, C. Review of ^{90}Y-ibritumomab tiuxetan as first-line consolidation radio-immunotherapy for B-cell follicular non-Hodgkin's lymphoma. *Cancer Manag. Res.* **2009**, *1*, 131–136. [CrossRef]
48. Mondello, P.; Cuzzocrea, S.; Navarra, M.; Mian, M. ^{90}Y-ibritumomab tiuxetan: A nearly forgotten opportunity. *Oncotarget* **2016**, *7*, 7597–7609. [CrossRef]
49. Ferrara, N.; Hillan, K.J.; Gerber, H.P.; Novotny, W. Discovery and development of bevacizumab, an anti-VEGF antibody for treating cancer. *Nat. Rev. Drug Discov.* **2004**, *3*, 391–400. [CrossRef]
50. Garcia, J.; Hurwitz, H.I.; Sandler, A.B.; Miles, D.; Coleman, R.L.; Deurloo, R.; Chinot, O.L. Bevacizumab (Avastin®) in cancer treatment: A review of 15 years of clinical experience and future outlook. *Cancer Treat. Rev.* **2020**, *86*. [CrossRef]
51. Jenkins, R.W.; Barbie, D.A.; Flaherty, K.T. Mechanisms of resistance to immune checkpoint inhibitors. *Br. J. Cancer* **2018**, *118*, 9–16. [CrossRef]
52. Darvin, P.; Toor, S.M.; Sasidharan Nair, V.; Elkord, E. Immune checkpoint inhibitors: Recent progress and potential biomarkers. *Exp. Mol. Med.* **2018**, *50*, 1–11. [CrossRef] [PubMed]
53. Mitsunaga, M.; Ogawa, M.; Kosaka, N.; Rosenblum, L.T.; Choyke, P.L.; Kobayashi, H. Cancer cell-selective in vivo near infrared photoimmunotherapy targeting specific membrane molecules. *Nat. Med.* **2011**, *17*, 1685–1691. [CrossRef]
54. Kobayashi, H.; Choyke, P.L. Near-infrared photoimmunotherapy of cancer. *Acc. Chem. Res.* **2019**, *52*, 2332–2339. [CrossRef]

55. Casalini, P.; Caldera, M.; Canevari, S.; Ménard, S.; Mezzanzanica, D.; Tosi, E.; Gadina, M.; Colnaghi, M.I. A critical comparison of three internalization assays applied to the evaluation of a given mAb as a toxin-carrier candidate. *Cancer Immunol. Immunother.* **1993**, *37*, 54–60. [CrossRef] [PubMed]
56. Liao-Chan, S.; Daine-Matsuoka, B.; Heald, N.; Wong, T.; Lin, T.; Cai, A.G.; Lai, M.; D'Alessio, J.A.; Theunissen, J.W. Quantitative assessment of antibody internalization with novel monoclonal antibodies against Alexa fluorophores. *PLoS ONE* **2015**, *10*. [CrossRef]
57. Li, Y.; Corbett Liu, P.; Shen, Y.; Snavely, M.D.; Hiraga, K. A cell-based internalization and degradation assay with an activatable fluorescence-quencher probe as a tool for functional antibody screening. *J. Biomol. Screen.* **2015**, *20*, 869–875. [CrossRef]
58. Rigo, A.; Vinante, F. Flow Cytometry analysis of receptor internalization/shedding. *Cytom. B* **2017**, *92B*, 291–298. [CrossRef] [PubMed]
59. Wargalla, U.C.; Reisfeld, R.A. Rate of internalization of an immunotoxin correlates with cytotoxic activity against human tumor cells. *Proc. Natl. Acad. Sci. USA* **1989**, *86*, 5146–5150. [CrossRef]
60. Sokolova, E.; Guryev, E.; Yudintsev, A.; Vodeneev, V.; Deyev, S.; Balalaeva, I. HER2-specific recombinant immunotoxin 4D5scFv-PE40 passes through retrograde trafficking route and forces cells to enter apoptosis. *Oncotarget* **2017**, *8*, 22048–22058. [CrossRef]
61. Derbyshire, E.J.; de Leij, L.; Wawrzynczak, E.J. Refinement of an indirect immunotoxin assay of monoclonal antibodies recognising the human small cell lung cancer cluster 2 antigen. *Br. J. Cancer* **1993**, *67*, 1242–1247. [CrossRef]
62. Weltman, J.K.; Pedroso, P.; Johnson, S.A.; Davignon, D.; Fast, L.D.; Leone, L.A. Rapid screening with indirect immunotoxin for monoclonal antibodies against human small cell lung cancer. *Cancer Res.* **1987**, *47*, 5552–5556.
63. Fukuhara, T.; Kim, J.; Hokaiwado, S.; Nawa, M.; Okamoto, H.; Kogiso, T.; Watabe, T.; Hattori, N. A novel immunotoxin reveals a new role for CD321 in endothelial cells. *PLoS ONE* **2017**, *12*. [CrossRef] [PubMed]
64. Awwad, S.; Angkawinitwong, U. Overview of Antibody Drug Delivery. *Pharmaceutics* **2018**, *10*, 83. [CrossRef]
65. Yamaguchi, M.; Nishii, Y.; Nakamura, K.; Aoki, H.; Hirai, S.; Uchida, H.; Sakuma, Y.; Hamada, H. Development of a sensitive screening method for selecting monoclonal antibodies to be internalized by cells. *Biochem. Biophys. Res. Commun.* **2014**, *454*, 600–603. [CrossRef]
66. Smith, G.P. Filamentous fusion phage: Novel expression vectors that display cloned antigens on the virion surface. *Science* **1985**, *228*, 1315–1317. [CrossRef]
67. Hou, S.C.; Chen, H.S.; Lin, H.W.; Chao, W.T.; Chen, Y.S.; Fu, C.Y.; Yu, C.M.; Huang, K.F.; Wang, A.H.; Yang, A.S. High throughput cytotoxicity screening of anti-HER2 immunotoxins conjugated with antibody fragments from phage-displayed synthetic antibody libraries. *Sci. Rep.* **2016**, *6*. [CrossRef]
68. Ledsgaard, L.; Kilstrup, M.; Karatt-Vellatt, A.; McCafferty, J.; Laustsen, A.H. Basics of antibody phage display technology. *Toxins* **2018**, *10*, 236. [CrossRef]
69. Babcook, J.S.; Leslie, K.B.; Olsen, O.A.; Salmon, R.A.; Schrader, J.W. A novel strategy for generating monoclonal antibodies from single, isolated lymphocytes producing antibodies of defined specificities. *Proc. Natl. Acad. Sci. USA* **1996**, *93*, 7843–7848. [CrossRef]
70. Tiller, T. Single B cell antibody technologies. *N. Biotechnol.* **2011**, *28*, 453–457. [CrossRef]
71. Drachman, J.G.; Senter, P.D. Antibody-drug conjugates: The chemistry behind empowering antibodies to fight cancer. *Hematol. Am. Soc. Hematol. Educ. Program.* **2013**, *2013*, 306–310. [CrossRef]
72. Beck, A.; Goetsch, L.; Dumontet, C.; Corvaïa, N. Strategies and challenges for the next generation of antibody–drug conjugates. *Nat. Rev. Drug Discov.* **2017**, *16*, 315–337. [CrossRef]
73. Hoffmann, R.M.; Coumbe, B.G.T.; Josephs, D.H.; Mele, S.; Ilieva, K.M.; Cheung, A.; Tutt, A.N.; Spicer, J.F.; Thurston, D.E.; Crescioli, S.; et al. Antibody structure and engineering considerations for the design and function of Antibody Drug Conjugates (ADCs). *Oncoimmunology* **2018**, *7*. [CrossRef]
74. Khongorzul, P.; Ling, C.J.; Khan, F.U.; Ihsan, A.U.; Zhang, J. Antibody–Drug Conjugates: A Comprehensive Review. *Mol. Cancer Res.* **2020**, *18*, 3–19. [CrossRef]
75. Pagano, L.; Fianchi, L.; Caira, M.; Rutella, S.; Leone, G. The role of Gemtuzumab Ozogamicin in the treatment of acute myeloid leukemia patients. *Oncogene* **2007**, *26*, 3679–3690. [CrossRef]
76. Kikkawa, Y.; Enomoto-Okawa, Y.; Fujiyama, A.; Fukuhara, T.; Harashima, N.; Sugawara, Y.; Negishi, Y.; Katagiri, F.; Hozumi, K.; Nomizu, M.; et al. Internalization of CD239 highly expressed in breast cancer cells: A potential antigen for antibody-drug conjugates. *Sci. Rep.* **2018**, *8*. [CrossRef]

77. Enomoto-Okawa, Y.; Maeda, Y.; Harashima, N.; Sugawara, Y.; Katagiri, F.; Hozumi, K.; Hui, K.M.; Nomizu, M.; Ito, Y.; Kikkawa, Y. An anti-human lutheran glycoprotein phage antibody inhibits cell migration on laminin-511: Epitope mapping of the antibody. *PLoS ONE* **2017**, *12*. [CrossRef]
78. Muguruma, K.; Yakushiji, F.; Kawamata, R.; Akiyama, D.; Arima, R.; Shirasaka, T.; Kikkawa, Y.; Taguchi, A.; Takayama, K.; Fukuhara, T.; et al. Novel hybrid compound of a plinabulin prodrug with an IgG binding peptide for generating a tumor selective noncovalent-type antibody-drug conjugate. *Bioconjugate Chem.* **2016**, *27*, 1606–1613. [CrossRef]
79. Nishii, Y.; Yamaguchi, M.; Kimura, Y.; Hasegawa, T.; Aburatani, H.; Uchida, H.; Hirata, K.; Sakuma, Y. A newly developed anti-Mucin 13 monoclonal antibody targets pancreatic ductal adenocarcinoma cells. *Int. J. Oncol.* **2015**, *46*, 1781–1787. [CrossRef]
80. Hamblett, K.J.; Senter, P.D.; Chace, D.F.; Sun, M.M.C.; Lenox, J.; Cerveny, C.G.; Kissler, K.M.; Bernhardt, S.X.; Kopcha, A.K.; Zabinski, R.F.; et al. Effects of drug loading on the antitumor activity of a monoclonal antibody drug conjugate. *Clin. Cancer Res.* **2004**, *10*, 7063–7070. [CrossRef]
81. Wakankar, A.; Chen, Y.; Gokarn, Y.; Jacobson, F.S. Analytical methods for physicochemical characterization of antibody drug conjugates. *mAbs* **2011**, *3*, 161–172. [CrossRef] [PubMed]
82. Ogitani, Y.; Aida, T.; Hagihara, K.; Yamaguchi, J.; Ishii, C.; Harada, N.; Soma, M.; Okamoto, H.; Oitate, M.; Arakawa, S.; et al. DS-8201a, A novel HER2-targeting ADC with a novel DNA topoisomerase I inhibitor, demonstrates a promising antitumor efficacy with differentiation from T-DM1. *Clin. Cancer Res.* **2016**, *22*, 5097–5108. [CrossRef] [PubMed]
83. Blanco, E.; Shen, H.; Ferrari, M. Principles of nanoparticle design for overcoming biological barriers to drug delivery. *Nat. Biotechnol.* **2015**, *33*, 941–951. [CrossRef] [PubMed]
84. Kumari, P.; Ghosh, B.; Biswas, S. Nanocarriers for cancer-targeted drug delivery. *J. Drug Target.* **2016**, *24*, 179–191. [CrossRef] [PubMed]
85. Allen, T.M.; Cullis, P.R. Liposomal drug delivery systems: From concept to clinical applications. *Adv. Drug Deliv. Rev.* **2013**, *65*, 36–48. [CrossRef] [PubMed]
86. Danhier, F. To exploit the tumor microenvironment: Since the EPR effect fails in the clinic, what is the future of nanomedicine? *J. Control. Release* **2016**, *244*, 108–121. [CrossRef] [PubMed]
87. Hare, J.I.; Lammers, T.; Ashford, M.B.; Puri, S.; Storm, G.; Barry, S.T. Challenges and strategies in anti-cancer nanomedicine development: An industry perspective. *Adv. Drug Deliv. Rev.* **2017**, *108*, 25–38. [CrossRef] [PubMed]
88. Krauss, A.C.; Gao, X.; Li, L.; Manning, M.L.; Patel, P.; Fu, W.; Janoria, K.G.; Gieser, G.; Bateman, D.A.; Przepiorka, D.; et al. FDA approval summary: (daunorubicin and cytarabine) liposome for injection for the treatment of adults with high-risk acute myeloid leukemia. *Clin. Cancer Res.* **2019**, *25*, 2685–2690. [CrossRef] [PubMed]
89. Trompetero, A.; Gordillo, A.; Del Pilar, M.C.; Cristina, V.M.; Bustos Cruz, R.H. Alzheimer's Disease and Parkinson's Disease: A Review of current treatment adopting a nanotechnology approach. *Curr. Pharm. Des.* **2018**, *24*, 22–45. [CrossRef] [PubMed]
90. Singh, A.P.; Biswas, A.; Shukla, A.; Maiti, P. Targeted therapy in chronic diseases using nanomaterial-based drug delivery vehicles. *Signal. Transduct. Target. Ther.* **2019**, *4*. [CrossRef] [PubMed]
91. Liu, X.; Madhankumar, A.B.; Miller, P.A.; Duck, K.A.; Hafenstein, S.; Rizk, E.; Slagle-Webb, B.; Sheehan, J.M.; Connor, J.R.; Yang, Q.X. MRI contrast agent for targeting glioma: Interleukin-13 labeled liposome encapsulating gadolinium-DTPA. *Neuro Oncol.* **2016**, *18*, 691–699. [CrossRef] [PubMed]
92. Suzuki, R.; Oda, Y.; Omata, D.; Nishiie, N.; Koshima, R.; Shiono, Y.; Sawaguchi, Y.; Unga, J.; Naoi, T.; Negishi, Y.; et al. Tumor growth suppression by the combination of nanobubbles and ultrasound. *Cancer Sci.* **2016**, *107*, 217–223. [CrossRef] [PubMed]
93. Ito, K.; Hamamichi, S.; Asano, M.; Hori, Y.; Matsui, J.; Iwata, M.; Funahashi, Y.; Umeda, I.O.; Fujii, H. Radiolabeled liposome imaging determines an indication for liposomal anticancer agent in ovarian cancer mouse xenograft models. *Cancer Sci.* **2016**, *107*, 60–67. [CrossRef]
94. Petersen, A.L.; Binderup, T.; Rasmussen, P.; Henriksen, J.R.; Elema, D.R.; Kjær, A.; Andresen, T.L. In vivo evaluation of PEGylated ^{64}Cu-liposomes with theranostic and radiotherapeutic potential using micro PET/CT. *Eur. J. Nucl. Med. Mol. Imaging* **2016**, *43*, 941–952. [CrossRef]
95. Koshkaryev, A.; Sawant, R.; Deshpande, M.; Torchilin, V. Immunoconjugates and long circulating systems: Origins, current state of the art and future directions. *Adv. Drug Deliv. Rev.* **2013**, *65*, 24–35. [CrossRef]

96. Eloy, J.O.; Petrilli, R.; Trevizan, L.N.F.; Chorilli, M. Immunoliposomes: A review on functionalization strategies and targets for drug delivery. *Colloids Surf. B Biointerfaces* **2017**, *159*, 454–467. [CrossRef]
97. Tran, S.; DeGiovanni, P.J.; Piel, B.; Rai, P. Cancer nanomedicine: A review of recent success in drug delivery. *Clin. Transl. Med.* **2017**, *6*. [CrossRef]
98. Park, J.W.; Hong, K.; Kirpotin, D.B.; Colbern, G.; Shalaby, R.; Baselga, J.; Shao, Y.; Nielsen, U.B.; Marks, J.D.; Moore, D.; et al. Anti-HER2 immunoliposomes: Enhanced efficacy attributable to targeted delivery. *Clin. Cancer Res.* **2002**, *8*, 1172–1181.
99. Eloy, J.O.; Petrilli, R.; Chesca, D.L.; Saggioro, F.P.; Lee, R.J.; Marchetti, J.M. Anti-HER2 immunoliposomes for co-delivery of paclitaxel and rapamycin for breast cancer therapy. *Eur. J. Pharm. Biopharm.* **2017**, *115*, 159–167. [CrossRef] [PubMed]
100. Vingerhoeds, M.H.; Steerenberg, P.A.; Hendriks, J.J.G.W.; Dekker, L.C.; van Hoesel, Q.G.C.M.; Crommelin, D.J.A.; Storm, S. Immunoliposome-mediated targeting of doxorubicin to human ovarian carcinoma in vitro and in vivo. *Br. J. Cancer* **1996**, *74*, 1023–1029. [CrossRef]
101. Dewhirst, M.W.; Secomb, T.W. Transport of drugs from blood vessels to tumour tissue. *Nat. Rev. Cancer* **2017**, *17*, 738–750. [CrossRef]
102. Dagogo-Jack, I.; Shaw, A.T. Tumour heterogeneity and resistance to cancer therapies. *Nat. Rev. Clin. Oncol.* **2018**, *15*, 81–94. [CrossRef]
103. Goldberg, M.S. Improving cancer immunotherapy through nanotechnology. *Nat. Rev. Cancer* **2019**, *19*, 587–602. [CrossRef]
104. Martin, J.D.; Cabral, H.; Stylianopoulos, T.; Jain, R.K. Improving cancer immunotherapy using nanomedicines: Progress, opportunities and challenges. *Nat. Rev. Clin. Oncol.* **2020**, *17*, 251–266. [CrossRef] [PubMed]
105. Vieira, D.B.; Gamarra, L.F. Getting into the brain: Liposome-based strategies for effective drug delivery across the blood-brain barrier. *Int. J. Nanomed.* **2016**, *11*, 5381–5414. [CrossRef] [PubMed]
106. Dong, X. Current strategies for brain drug delivery. *Theranostics* **2018**, *8*, 1481–1493. [CrossRef]
107. Villaseñor, R.; Lampe, J.; Schwaninger, M.; Collin, L. Intracellular transport and regulation of transcytosis across the blood–brain barrier. *Cell. Mol. Life Sci.* **2019**, *76*, 1081–1092. [CrossRef] [PubMed]
108. Pulgar, V.M. Transcytosis to cross the blood brain barrier, new advancements and challenges. *Front. Neurosci.* **2019**, *12*, 1019. [CrossRef] [PubMed]
109. Johnsen, K.B.; Burkhart, A.; Melander, F.; Kempen, P.J.; Vejlebo, J.B.; Siupka, P.; Nielsen, M.S.; Andresen, T.L.; Moos, T. Targeting transferrin receptors at the blood-brain barrier improves the uptake of immunoliposomes and subsequent cargo transport into the brain parenchyma. *Sci. Rep.* **2017**, *7*. [CrossRef]
110. Zhang, Y.; Schlachetzki, F.; Pardridge, W.M. Global non-viral gene transfer to the primate brain following intravenous administration. *Mol. Ther.* **2003**, *7*, 11–18. [CrossRef]
111. Boado, R.J.; Pardridge, W.M. The trojan horse liposome technology for nonviral gene transfer across the blood-brain barrier. *J. Drug Deliv.* **2011**. [CrossRef] [PubMed]

toxins

MDPI

Article

Primary Sequence and 3D Structure Prediction of the Plant Toxin Stenodactylin

Rosario Iglesias [1,†], Letizia Polito [2,†], Massimo Bortolotti [2], Manuela Pedrazzi [2], Lucía Citores [1], José M. Ferreras [1,*] and Andrea Bolognesi [2,*]

1. Department of Biochemistry and Molecular Biology and Physiology, Faculty of Sciences, University of Valladolid, E−47011 Valladolid, Spain; riglesia@bio.uva.es (R.I.); luciac@bio.uva.es (L.C.)
2. Department of Experimental, Diagnostic and Specialty Medicine—DIMES, General Pathology Section, Alma Mater Studiorum—University of Bologna, Via S. Giacomo 14, 40126 Bologna, Italy; letizia.polito@unibo.it (L.P.); massimo.bortolotti2@unibo.it (M.B.); manuela_pedrazzi@hotmail.com (M.P.)

* Correspondence: josemiguel.ferreras@uva.es (J.M.F.); andrea.bolognesi@unibo.it (A.B.)

† These authors contributed equally to this work.

Received: 23 July 2020; Accepted: 19 August 2020; Published: 21 August 2020

Abstract: Stenodactylin is one of the most potent type 2 ribosome-inactivating proteins (RIPs); its high toxicity has been demonstrated in several models both in vitro and in vivo. Due to its peculiarities, stenodactylin could have several medical and biotechnological applications in neuroscience and cancer treatment. In this work, we report the complete amino acid sequence of stenodactylin and 3D structure prediction. The comparison between the primary sequence of stenodactylin and other RIPs allowed us to identify homologies/differences and the amino acids involved in RIP toxic activity. Stenodactylin RNA was isolated from plant caudex, reverse transcribed through PCR and the cDNA was amplificated and cloned into a plasmid vector and further analyzed by sequencing. Nucleotide sequence analysis showed that stenodactylin A and B chains contain 251 and 258 amino acids, respectively. The key amino acids of the active site described for ricin and most other RIPs are also conserved in the stenodactylin A chain. Stenodactylin amino acid sequence shows a high identity degree with volkensin (81.7% for A chain, 90.3% for B chain), whilst when compared with other type 2 RIPs the identity degree ranges from 27.7 to 33.0% for the A chain and from 42.1 to 47.7% for the B chain.

Keywords: 3D structure; plant toxin; primary sequence; ribosome-inactivating protein; stenodactylin; toxic lectin

Key Contribution: The complete amino acid sequence and 3D structure prediction of stenodactylin are essential because of their potential medical and biotechnological applications in neuroscience and cancer treatment.

---

1. Introduction

Ribosome-inactivating proteins (RIPs) are a family of enzymes widely spread throughout the plant kingdom. RIPs are found in different angiosperms and are also present in some fungal and bacterial species [1]. Many RIP-producing plants have been used for centuries in traditional medicine, and they are still used in folk medicine against several pathologies [2,3]. RIPs possess rRNA N-glycosilase and polynucleotide: adenosine glycosilase activities; RIPs are able to remove one or more adenine from rRNA and several other polynucleotide substrates, thus causing ribosome damage and cell death [1,4,5]. Based on their structure, RIPs are divided into two main groups: type 1 and type 2. The first group consists of RIPs characterized by a single polypeptide chain, of about 30 kDa, with enzymatic activity. The second group includes toxins, with molecular weight of 60–65 kDa, consisting of two polypeptide chains: an enzymatically active A-chain, with properties similar to type 1 RIPs, linked through a disulfide bond to a B-chain with lectin properties. The B-chain has strong affinity for sugar moieties on the cell surface and can facilitate the entry of the toxin into the cell, thus conferring to many type 2 RIPs high cytotoxic effect [6].

Amongst type 2 RIPs, one of the most potent is stenodactylin, purified from the caudex of *Adenia stenodactyla* Harms, a tropical plant belonging to the Passifloraceae family. This RIP has a high enzymatic activity toward ribosomes and herring sperm DNA substrates and is specific for galactose [7]. Interestingly, stenodactylin showed a very low median lethal dose for mice, 2.76 μg/kg at 48 h [7], comparable or lower than the LD_{50}s reported in the literature for ricin, ranging from 2 to 22 μg/kg [6].

Like other RIPs purified from *Adenia* species, namely, modeccin and volkensin [8], stenodactylin is retrogradely transported when injected into the central nervous system [9]. This property could have several medical and biotechnological applications in the field of neuroscience to selectively lesion specific neurons.

It has been reported that in a neuroblastoma cell line, stenodactylin can induce multiple cell death pathways, involving mainly apoptosis, but also necroptosis and the production of free radicals [10]. Similar results have been recently obtained in acute myeloid leukemia cells, in which stenodactylin can elicit a rapid stress response with production of pro-inflammatory factors and oxidative stress leading mainly to apoptosis, but also triggering other cell death pathways [11].

RIPs have been studied for many years because of their therapeutic use as toxic moieties of immunotoxins, chimeric molecules obtained conjugating a cytotoxic RIP to a specific carrier, mainly a monoclonal antibody, thus allowing for the selective killing of target cells. Immunotoxins have been included in several clinical trials against various diseases, often achieving promising results, especially in the treatment of hematological neoplasms [12,13]. Due to its high cytotoxic potential, stenodactylin could represent an ideal candidate both as toxic moiety of immunotoxins for the treatment of cancers, and as a single agent for loco-regional treatments. In order to envisage such uses, the knowledge of the primary sequence of stenodactylin and the comparison with the amino acid sequence of other RIPs are essential, thus providing useful information about cell interaction and the toxicity mechanism of stenodactylin.

Through comparing amino acid sequences of RIPs, a high similarity can be observed between type 1 and the A chains of type 2 RIPs and among the B chains of type 2 RIPs. However, the primary structure homologies can vary from 15 to 80% between RIPs from different species [14]. X-ray diffraction analyses showed that the 3D-structures of RIPs are well conserved, with differences in the only C-terminal region and the surface loop structure. Ricin was the first RIP to be analyzed by X-ray diffraction. Ricin A chain is a globular protein that is folded into three domains that largely exhibit α-helical and β-strand structures [15]. The A chain includes two N-glycosylation sites (Asn10-Phe11-Thr12 and Asn236-Gly237-Ser238), but these sites do not appear to be important for proper folding [16]. Ricin B chain consists of two topologically similar domains (lectins), composed by four subdomains (1λ, 1α, 1β and 1γ for domain 1 and 2λ, 2α, 2β and 2γ for domain 2). Only 1α and 2γ subdomains demonstrated galactose-binding activity through a network of hydrogen bonds [15].

Crystallization and preliminary X-ray diffraction data analyses of stenodactylin have already been reported [17], but very little is known about the protein sequence level. Only the first 22 and 21 amino acid residues of the A and B chains have been determined using direct Edman degradation. A protein sequence alignment between stenodactylin, modeccin (*A. digitata*), lanceolin A1, lanceolin A2 (*A. lanceolata*) and volkensin (*A. volkensii*) showed that the A chain of stenodactylin shares 21/21 identity with lanceolin A2 and 15/21 with volkensin. The identity among the B chains is also very high, except for the first three N-terminal residues; the sequence Asp-Pro-Valis present only in the stenodactylin and volkensin B chains [7].

In this work we report the complete amino acid sequence of stenodactylin. The comparison of the stenodactylin primary sequence with that of the other RIPs and the homology degree allowed us to identify the amino acids directly or indirectly involved in RIP toxicity.

2. Results

2.1. *Stenodactylin Gene Sequence*

Based on of the N-terminal amino acid sequences of the A and B chains of stenodactylin previously obtained by Edman degradation [7] and based on the amino acid sequence of volkensin (CAD61022), five specific primers were designed for the PCR amplification of stenodactylin cDNA (see Section 4.2.1). Three primer pairs were used to amplify the A chain (STA2-STB1R), the A chain with part of the B chain (STA2-STB3R) and the B chain (STB1-STB5R) of stenodactylin. The fragments corresponding to the stenodactylin gene ends presented a homologous overlapping region. The sequence information was analyzed using the algorithms available at http://expasy.org [18]. Excluding the nucleotide sequence coding for the signal peptide, the full-length caudex cDNA sequence analysis revealed that stenodactylin is encoded by a 1572-bp open reading frame (ORF) that encoded a polypeptide of 524 amino acids (Figure 1). Only the first 11 amino acids were obtained exclusively by Edman degradation.

```
nnnnnnnnnnnnnnnnnnnnnnnnnnnnnnnnnnnngccacggtagagaggtacactcagttt   60
 V  F  P  K  V  I  F  D  C  T  R  A  T  V  E  R  Y  T  Q  F    20
ataatgctcttaaggaacgaactggcgggtgatgtttctccacagggaatacgcaggctg  120
 I  M  L  L  R  N  E  L  A  G  D  V  S  P  Q  G  I  R  R  L    40
aggaatccggctgatattcagcctacacagcgttttattcttatacaactcaacggcttc  180
 R  N  P  A  D  I  Q  P  T  Q  R  F  I  L  I  Q  L  N  G  F    60
gtaagctccgtcaccttgataatggacgtcagcaatgcgtatctattgggttatgagagc  240
 V  S  S  V  T  L  I  M  D  V  S  N  A  Y  L  L  G  Y  E  S    80
cgcaactttgtgtatcacttcaacgatgtctctacctcttcgatcgccgatgttttccca  300
 R  N  F  V  Y  H  F  N  D  V  S  T  S  S  I  A  D  V  F  P   100
gacgtacaacgtcaacagttgccatttgaaggcggctatcccagcatgcgacactatgcg  360
 D  V  Q  R  Q  Q  L  P  F  E  G  G  Y  P  S  M  R  H  Y  A   120
ccggagagagatcaaattgaccatggattcatcgaactggcatacgctgttgatacgctc  420
 P  E  R  D  Q  I  D  H  G  F  I  E  L  A  Y  A  V  D  T  L   140
[illegible]
 Y  Y  S  S  Q  G  Y  E  Q  I  A  R  S  L  V  L  C  A  G  M   160
gttgcagaagccgcccggttccgctacatcgaggggctagtgcgtcaaagcattgtcggg  540
 V  A  E  A  A  R  F  R  Y  I  E  G  L  V  R  Q  S  I  V  G   180
ccaggagactacggaactttcagaccggatgcgttgatgtactcagtcgtgacagcgtgg  600
 P  G  D  Y  G  T  F  R  P  D  A  L  M  Y  S  V  V  T  A  W   200
cagactctttcagaaagaatccagggatccttcgacggagctttccagccagttcagctg  660
 Q  T  L  S  E  R  I  Q  G  S  F  D  G  A  F  Q  P  V  Q  L   220
gggtatgccagcgatcccttttattgggacaacgtcgcacaggccatcaccaggctgtca  720
 G  Y  A  S  D  P  F  Y  W  D  N  V  A  Q  A  I  T  R  L  S   240
ctcatgctattcgcctgcgctaaacctccaaggcaatccgattccctcatggtgataagg  780
 L  M  L  F  A  C  A  K  P  P  R  Q  S  D  S  L  M  V  I  R   251
tcctttgtggataggaacgatcctgtctgcccttccggggagacgactgcgtacatcgtg  840
 S  F  V  D  R  N  D  P  V  C  P  S  G  E  T  T  A  Y  I  V    14
gggcgggacgggcgctgtgtggacgtgaaggatgaggaattcttcgacggcaataaagta  900
 G  R  D  G  R  C  V  D  V  K  D  E  E  F  F  D  G  N  K  V    34
cagatgtggccgtgcaagtccagccagaatgcaaaccagctgtggactataaagagagac  960
 Q  M  W  P  C  K  S  S  Q  N  A  N  Q  L  W  T  I  K  R  D    54
ggcactattcggtgcaagggaaagtgcttgactgtgaggagcccgcaactgtacgctatg 1020
 G  T  I  R  C  K  G  K  C  L  T  V  R  S  P  Q  L  Y  A  M    74
atctgggactgcaccacttttatgctcctgccaccaagtgggaagtgtgggacaacggg 1080
 I  W  D  C  T  T  F  Y  A  P  A  T  K  W  E  V  W  D  N  G    94
accatcatcaaccccgcctccgggagggtgttgaccgcgcccactggggacgcgggcgtc 1140
 T  I  I  N  P  A  S  G  R  V  L  T  A  P  T  G  D  A  G  V   114
atcctcagcctggagctcaacgagtacgccgctagccaggcgtggagggtgaccaatgtg 1200
 I  L  S  L  E  L  N  E  Y  A  A  S  Q  A  W  R  V  T  N  V   134
acagtacctacggtggcaaccattgtgggatatgatgatctctgcctggaaaccaacgac 1260
 T  V  P  T  V  A  T  I  V  G  Y  D  D  L  C  L  E  T  N  D   154
aacaatgtatggttggtcaactgcgtgaaaggcaagacgcaacagagatgggcgcagtat 1320
 N  N  V  W  L  V  N  C  V  K  G  K  T  Q  Q  R  W  A  Q  Y   174
gcggatggcaccatacgctcccagtccagcctcagcaaatgcctcacctgcagtggcgac 1380
 A  D  G  T  I  R  S  Q  S  S  L  S  K  C  L  T  C  S  G  D   194
tgcgtcaagctggcaaagatcgtcaacacggactgtgctggatccgccttgagccgttgg 1440
 C  V  K  L  A  K  I  V  N  T  D  C  A  G  S  A  L  S  R  W   214
tacttcaacacctatggcggcatcgtgaatctgttgaccggcatggtgatggacgtgaaa 1500
 Y  F  N  T  Y  G  G  I  V  N  L  L  T  G  M  V  M  D  V  K   234
gagtccaatccgagtctcaacgaaataattgcccacccgtggcatggaaactccaaccag 1560
 E  S  N  P  S  L  N  E  I  I  A  H  P  W  H  G  N  S  N  Q   254
caatggttccta 1572
 Q  W  F  L   258
```

Figure 1. Full length sequence and derived amino acid sequence of the stenodactylin gene. The A chain is presented in black; the B chain is presented in blue and the sequence of the connecting peptides is presented in red. The amino acid sequences obtained by Edman degradation, as described in [7], are underlined. Numbering refers to the position of the amino acids in the mature A and B chains. The cDNA sequence for stenodactylin was submitted to GenBank (accession number: MT580807). The letter "n" means "unknown nucleotide residue", being the amino acid sequence obtained exclusively by Edman degradation.

The gene contains 753 bp that encode the A chain (251 amino acid residues with a calculated relative molecular mass (Mr) of 28,420.32) and 774 bp that encode the B chain (258 amino acid residues with a calculated Mr of 28,567.34) separated by a sequence of 45 bp that encodes the connecting peptide (Figure 1). The probable C-terminal end of the A chain and the connecting peptide were estimated based on the homology with volkensin.

Stenodactylin contains a total of 15 cysteine residues. The A chain includes Cys9, Cys157 and the C-terminal Cys246, which is involved in the intermolecular disulfide bond. The B chain includes 12 cysteines (Cys4, Cys20, Cys39, Cys59, Cys63, Cys78, Cys149, Cys162, Cys188, Cys191, Cys195, Cys206), eight of which (Cys20-Cys39, Cys63-Cys78, Cys149-Cys162, and Cys188-Cys206) form conserved intramolecular disulfide bridges; one cysteine (Cys4) at the N-terminal binds to the A chain. The amino acid residues that are important for the enzymatic activity of RIPs were conserved within the sequence of the A chain of stenodactylin (Tyr74, Tyr113, Glu163, Arg166, and Trp200).

In addition, based on the online program NetNGlyc1.0 [19], two possible glycosylation sites were detected at position Asn93-Gly94-Thr95 and Asn133-Val134-Thr135 in the B chain. This is noteworthy because, although N-glycosylation does not affect the catalytic activity of RIPs, it can affect their intracellular routing, their cytotoxicity and their immunogenicity [20,21].

Based on the amino acid sequence, the secondary structure was predicted by the highly accurate PSIPRED algorithm for protein secondary structure prediction [22]. The 509 amino acid-long protein was calculated to have 25.7% extended strands, 21.6% α helices and 52.7% random coils, with α-helix structures mainly present in the A chain (Figure 2).

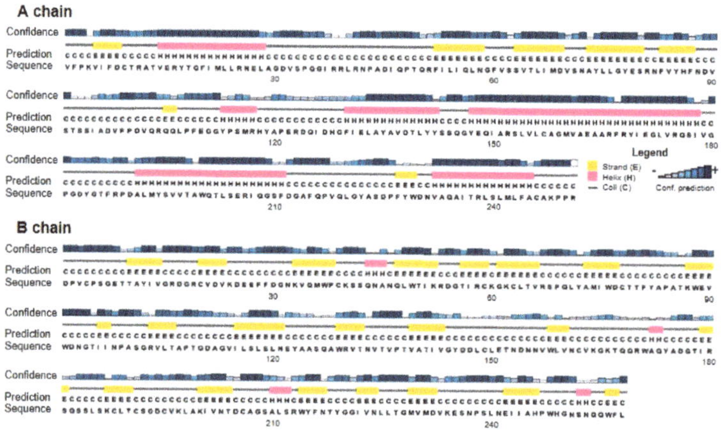

Figure 2. Secondary structure analysis of stenodactylin A and B chains. The secondary structure motifs were predicted using the PSIPRED Protein Structure Prediction Server. The predicted helix (H, pink) and strand (E, yellow) structure elements and randomly structured coil regions (C) of the target sequences are displayed according to the symbols shown in the legend. The confidence levels of the prediction are reported in the figure.

The stenodactylin polypeptide sequence was aligned with volkensin using the Clustal Omega software [23]. A comparison of the amino acid sequence of stenodactylin with volkensin showed

86.1% amino acid identity (Figure 3). This homology was not surprising because these two RIPs were purified from plants belonging to the same genus (*Adenia*). The results show higher identity between the B chains (90.3%) than between the A chains (81.7%). In addition, the A chain of stenodactylin contains one more cysteine at position 9 compared with volkensin. The B chains of both stenodactylin and volkensin contain 12 cysteine residues.

The catalytic key residues that are involved in the enzymatic mechanism and the 25 amino acids that are involved in the active center of the A chain (Figure 3) are almost conserved, except for Ala199 and Ala245, in stenodactylin, which are replaced with Gln198 and Val244, in volkensin.

```
VOLKENSIN     VFPKVPFDVPKATVESYTRFIRVLRDELAGGVSPQGIRRLRNPAEIQPSQGFILIQLTGY  60
STENODACTYLIN VFPKVIFDCTRATVERYTQFIMLLRNELAGDVSPQGIRRLRNPADIQPTQRFILIQLNGF  60
              ***** **   :**** **:** :**:**** *************:***:* ******.*:

VOLKENSIN     VGSVTLIMDVRNAYLLGYLSHNVLYHFNDVSASSIASVFPDAQRRQLPFGGGYPSMRNYA 120
STENODACTYLIN VSSVTLIMDVSNAYLLGYESRNFVYHFNDVSTSSIADVFPDVQRQQLPFEGGYPSMRHYA 120
              *.******** ******* *:*.:*******:****.****.**:**** *******.**

VOLKENSIN     PERDQIDHGIVELAYAVDRLYYSQ-NNNQIALGLVICAGMVAEASRFRYIEGLVRQSIVG 179
STENODACTYLIN PERDQIDHGFIELAYAVDTLYYSSQGYEQIARSLVLCAGMVAEAARFRYIEGLVRQSIVG 180
              *********::******* ****.     :*** .**:********:***************

VOLKENSIN     PGDYRTFRPDALMYSIVTQWQTLSERIQGSFNGAFQPVQLGYASDPFYWDNVAQAITRLS 239
STENODACTYLIN PGDYGTFRPDALMYSVVTAWQTLSERIQGSFDGAFQPVQLGYASDPFYWDNVAQAITRLS 240
              **** **********:** ************:*****************************

VOLKENSIN     LMLFVCSQPPRQSDSPLVIRSFVDRNDPVCPSGETTAFIVGRDGRCVDVKVEEFFDGNKV  34
STENODACTYLIN LMLFACAKPPRQSDSLMVIRSFVDRNDPVCPSGETTAYIVGRDGRCVDVKDEEFFDGNKV  34
              ****.*::******* :*********************:************ *********

VOLKENSIN     QMWPCKSSQNANQLWTLKRDGTIRCQGKCLTVRSPQLYAMIWDCTTFYAPATKWEVWDNG  94
STENODACTYLIN QMWPCKSSQNANQLWTIKRDGTIRCKGKCLTVRSPQLYAMIWDCTTFYAPATKWEVWDNG  94
              ****************:*********:**********************************
VOLKENSIN     TIINPASGRVLTAPTGEAGVTLNLQFNEYAASQAWRVTNVTVPTVTTIVGYDDLCLETNG 154
STENODACTYLIN TIINPASGGVLTAPTGDAGVILSLELNEYAASQAWRVTNVTVPTVATIVGYDDLCLETND 154
              ******** *******:*** *.*::********************:*************

VOLKENSIN     NGVWLANCVKGKAQQRWTLYADGTIRSQSTLSKCLACSGSCVKLAKIVNTDCAGSANSRW 214
STENODACTYLIN NNVWLVNCVKGKTQQRWAQYADGTIRSQSSLSKCLTCSGDCVKLAKIVNTDCAGSALSRW 214
              * ***.******:****: **********:*****:***.**************** ***

VOLKENSIN     YFDNYGGIVNLRTGMVMDVKESNPSLNEIIAHPWHGNSNQQWFL 258
STENODACTYLIN YFNTYGGIVNLLTGMVMDVKESNPSLNEIIAHPWHGNSNQQWFL 258
              **:.******* ********************************
```

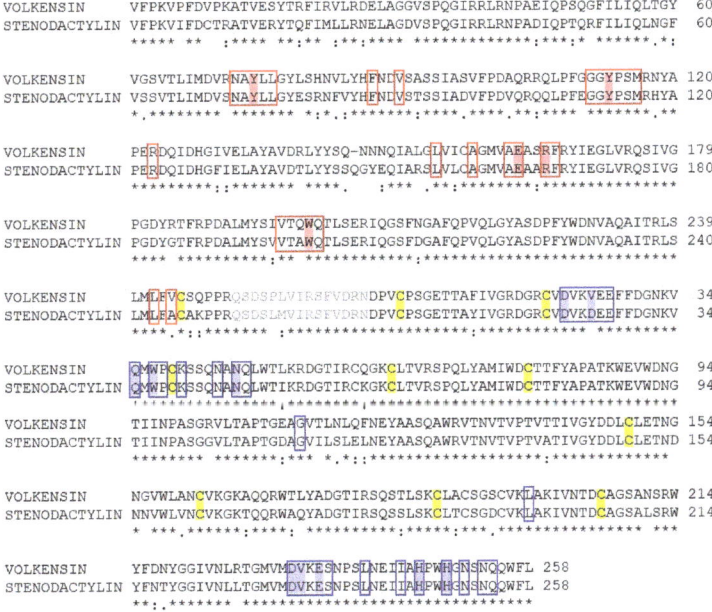

Figure 3. Alignment between stenodactylin and volkensin (GenBank CAD61022). Identical residues (*), conserved substitutions (:) and semiconserved substitutions (.) are reported. The A and B chains are presented in black; the sequence of the linker peptides is presented in gray. The putative amino acids that are present in the active site pocket (boxed in red) or in the galactoside-binding sites (boxed in blue), those involved in substrate binding or catalysis (highlighted in red), those involved in sugar binding (highlighted in blue), and those involved in disulfide bridges (highlighted in yellow) are represented, and they were assigned by comparison with the structure of ricin (accession no. 2AAI, 3RTI and 3RTJ). The dash indicates a gap introduced into the sequences to maximize alignments.

2.2. Structure of Stenodactylin

To ascertain the main structural characteristics of stenodactylin, a three-dimensional structure was predicted by comparative modelling using several type 2 RIP crystal structures as templates. The selected best model was found to have a confidence score (C-score) of 0.64, template modelling (Tm) score of 0.80 ± 0.09, and root-mean-square deviation (RMSD) of 6.0 ± 3.7 Å, which satisfied the range of parameters for molecular modelling.

Even though stenodactylin shares a low amino acid sequence identity with both ricin and abrin-a (Table 1), it has a 3D structure similar to that of ricin [24] and abrin-a [25] (Figure 4, Figure S2). Stenodactylin is formed by a 251 amino acid A-chain bound to a B-chain of 258 amino acids by a disulfide bond in which Cys246 of the A chain and Cys4 of the B-chain participate.

Table 1. Identity of eight type 2 RIPs and three type 1 RIPs with stenodactylin.

	RIP Name	Identity (%) Stenodactylin A Chain	Identity (%) Stenodactylin B Chain	Identity (%) Stenodactylin Whole Molecule
Type 2	Volkensin	81.7	90.3	86.1
	Ricin	31.4	47.7	40.3
	Viscumin	31.0	46.0	38.1
	Abrin a	31.2	44.6	37.9
	Riproximin	27.7	43.3	35.8
	Cinnamomin	33.0	42.1	37.3
	Ebulin l	28.7	44.2	36.5
	Nigrin b	29.0	43.9	36.5
Type 1	Saporin	18.9		
	Dianthin	18.1		
	Momordin	24.0		

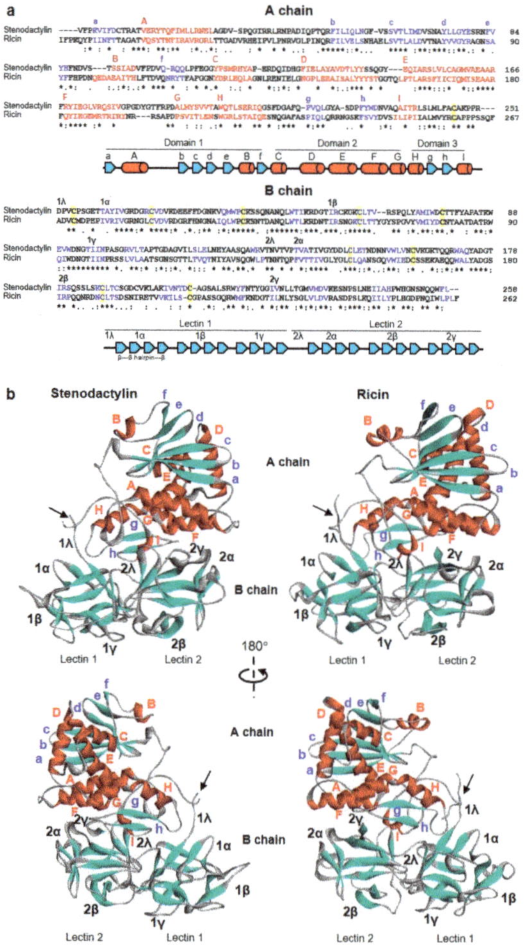

Figure 4. Structure of stenodactylin compared with ricin. (**a**) Amino acid sequence alignment of the A and B chains of stenodactylin and ricin. The β strands (blue), the α helices (red) and the cysteines

involved in the disulfide bonds (highlighted in yellow) are indicated. The helices are labelled A to I and the strands of the β sheets are labelled a to h in the A chain. The domains and subdomains in the B chain are also indicated. Identical residues (*), conserved substitutions (:) and semiconserved substitutions (.) are reported. The cartoons represent the different structural motifs in both A and B chains. (**b**) Three-dimensional structure of stenodactylin compared with ricin (Protein Data Bank accession no. 2AAI). The three-dimensional structural modelling was carried out on the I-TASSER server and the figure was generated using Discovery Studio 2016. The α helices (red), the β chains (cyan), and the coils (grey) are represented. The helices are labelled A to I and the strands of the β sheets are labelled a to h in the A chain. The structural domains and subdomains in the B chain are also indicated. Arrows indicate the position of the disulfide bond linking A and B chains.

The A chain can be divided into three folding domains that come together creating a deep active site pocket. This is common, not only to A-chains of type 2 RIPs but also to type 1 RIPs [26]. Domain 1 extends from the N-terminus to residue 109 and consists of six β-strands (strands a to f) and two α-helices (helices A and B) alternating in the order aAbcdeBf (Figure 4a). The six β-strands are arranged in a β-sheet of antiparallel strands sitting on domain 2 (Figure 4b). In domain 1, the Tyr74 that participates in the binding of adenine is located. Domain 2 is composed of residues from 110 to 199 and consists of five α-helices (C–G helices) containing the catalytic amino acids Glu163 and Arg166 and the other amino acid that binds adenine (Tyr113). Domain 3 extends from residue 200 to the C-terminus and consists of an α-helix-β-fork-α-helix (HghI) motif that is characteristic of A chains of type 2 RIPs and type 1 RIPs derived from type 2 RIPs by B-chain deletion. This structural motif has been related to the ability of these proteins to cross membranes [26] and contains the Trp200 that closes the active site.

Stenodactylin B-chain is composed of two homologous lectins, each of them consisting of four subdomains, λ, α, β and γ (Figure 4a). Subdomain 1λ (residues 1 to 9) participates in the disulfide bonding of the A- and B-chains and subdomain 2λ (residues 131 to 137) connects the two lectins of the B-chain. Lectin 1 contains the homologous subdomains 1α (residues 10 to 56), 1β (residues 57 to 94) and 1γ (residues 95 to 130), which are organized in a β trefoil fold. Each subdomain consists of a β-strand, a β-fork, and another β-strand. The β-strands form a six-strand β-barrel and the three β-forks form a lid on the barrel (Figure 4b, Figure 5). This structure is repeated in lectin 2 with subdomains 2α (residues 138 to 178), 2β (179 to 221) and 2γ (221 to 258). The central structure of the β-strands of lectins 1 and 2 is very similar in stenodactylin and ricin, while the main differences are found in the loops that stand out from these central structures (Figure 4b).

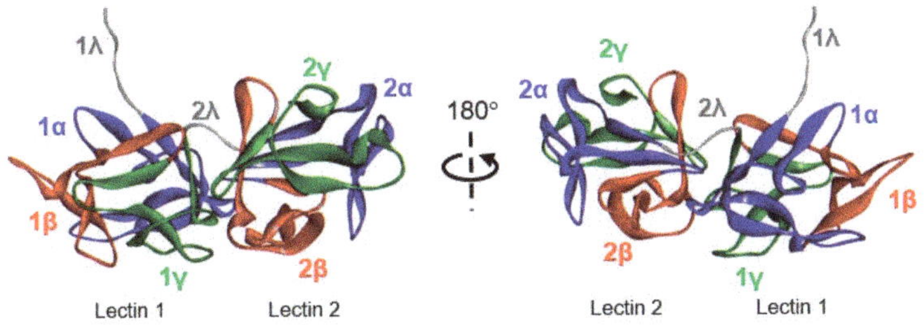

Figure 5. Structure of stenodactylin B chain. The three-dimensional structural modelling was carried out on the I-TASSER server and the figure was generated using Discovery Studio 2016. The structural domains and subdomains in the B chain are indicated.

2.3. Sequence Comparison between Stenodactylin and Other RIPs

The sequence of stenodactylin was aligned and compared with the sequences of other RIPs, including both type 2 (toxic and non-toxic) and type 1.

The alignment and comparison are important (i) to identify both conserved and non-conserved amino acids, (ii) to understand the degree of evolutionary change and (iii) to detect amino acids that are important for their enzymatic activity.

The amino acid sequence of stenodactylin was aligned with the amino acid sequences of toxic type 2 RIPs (e.g., volkensin, ricin, abrin, viscumin, riproximin) and non-toxic (e.g., cinnamomin, ebulin l and nigrin b) that have been reported in GenBank (Table 1, Figure 6). The multiple alignment analysis showed that, in all RIP evaluated, the B chains contain eight cysteine residues, involved in four conserved intramolecular disulfide bridges, and the B chain N-terminal cysteine that forms the intermolecular disulfide bridge between the A and B chains. Furthermore, the catalytic key residues (Tyr74, Tyr113, Glu163, Arg166, Trp200 in stenodactylin) that are involved in the enzymatic mechanism and the binding of adenine are conserved in all A chains of the RIPs.

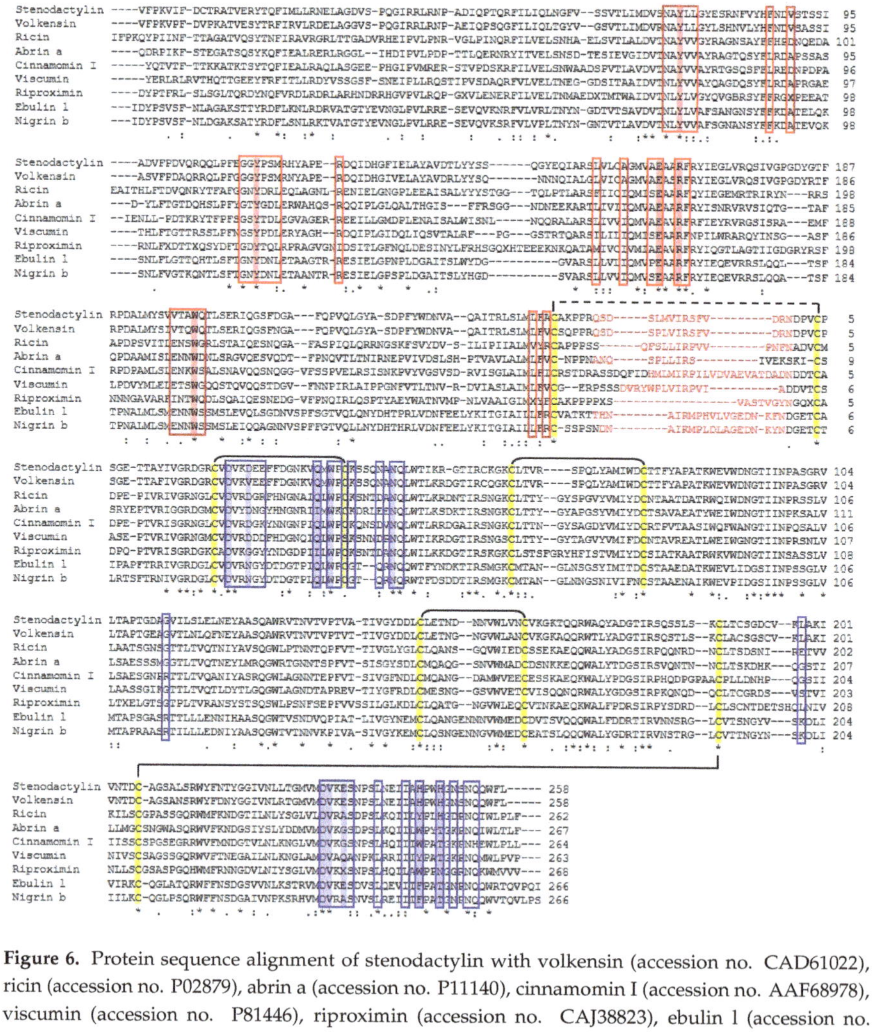

Figure 6. Protein sequence alignment of stenodactylin with volkensin (accession no. CAD61022), ricin (accession no. P02879), abrin a (accession no. P11140), cinnamomin I (accession no. AAF68978), viscumin (accession no. P81446), riproximin (accession no. CAJ38823), ebulin l (accession no. CAC33178), and nigrin b (accession no. P33183). Identical residues (*), conserved substitutions (:) and semiconserved substitutions (.) are reported. The A and B chains are presented in black and the sequence of the connecting peptide is presented in red. The putative amino acids that are present in the

active site pocket (boxed in red) or in the galactoside-binding sites (boxed in blue), those involved in substrate binding or catalysis (highlighted in red), those involved in sugar binding (highlighted in blue), and those involved in disulphide bridges (highlighted in yellow) are represented, and they were assigned by comparison with the structure of ricin (accession no. 2AAI, 3RTI and 3RTJ). Dashes denote gaps introduced into the sequences to maximize alignments.

Table 1 reports the identity between stenodactylin with toxic and non-toxic type 2 RIPs and type 1 RIPs. The results show that there is a high percentage of identity between the A and B chains of stenodactylin and volkensin. All other identities were lower, ranging from 27.7 to 33.0% for A chains and from 42.1 to 47.7% for B chains. The identity with type 1 RIPs is very low, being 18.1, 18.9 and 24.0% with dianthin, saporin and momordin, respectively.

The sequence of A- and B-chains of stenodactylin compared with the logos of type 2 RIPs from 28 plant species are shown in Figure 7. These logos are representative of all type 2 RIPs of the plant kingdom as each species is represented by one, two or three sequences. The A chain is the least conserved, but still has 24 almost invariable amino acids (with a frequency greater than 90%). Four of these amino acids are located in the active site (Tyr143, Glu201, Arg204 and Trp241 of the logo, which correspond to the residues Tyr113, Glu163, Arg166, and Trp200 of stenodactylin). It is worth mentioning that residue 98 in the active site is frequently (83%) Tyr (Tyr74 in stenodactylin), but it may be replaced by other amino acids. Ser245 (204 in stenodactylin) is not in the active site but is adjacent to and stabilizes the Trp of the active site. The other invariant amino acids are located outside and away from the active site and it has been postulated that they could participate in the internal dynamics of the enzyme [26]. Stenodactylin has two changes in these amino acids (Pro57 and Ala291 in the logo are Arg38 and Ser240 in stenodactylin, respectively).

The B chain is much more conserved (Figure 7) and has 52 amino acids with a frequency greater than 90%, and only changes Leu116 by Arg103 in stenodactylin. Some of these amino acids are located in the 1α (Asp27, Val28, Asn51, Gln52 that correspond to residues 22, 23, 46 and 47 of stenodactylin) and 2γ (Asp268, Val269, Leu276, Gln291 which correspond to residues 232, 233, 240 and 254 of stenodactylin) sites, but most of them are outside and even away from sugar binding sites. It has been suggested that these amino acids could complete the symmetry of both β trefoils or could constitute a structure that expands from the 1α site to the 2γ site participating in a network of protein motions that functionally connect both sugar binding sites [26]. Finally, it should be mentioned that only four amino acids directly involved in the binding of sugars (Asp27 and Asn51 in the 1α site, Asp268 and Val269 in the 2γ site) are highly conserved.

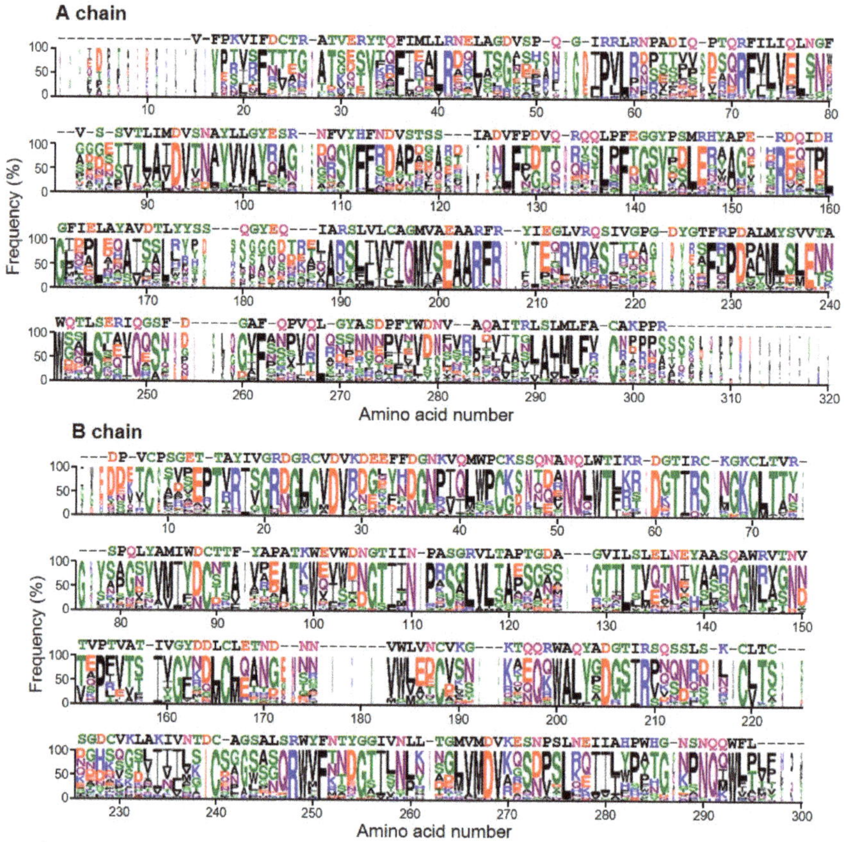

Figure 7. Sequence logos of the A and B chains of type 2 RIPs. The sequence logo representation of the alignment of the A and B-chain sequences from 46 representative type 2 RIPs belonging to 28 plant species was created as indicated in the "Materials and Methods" section. Letter height is proportional to the frequency of that amino acid at that position in the alignment respect to all the amino acids; letter width is proportional to the frequency of that amino acid but includes gaps. The sequence of stenodactylin is indicated above the logos.

2.4. Phylogenetic Analysis

To understand the relationship between stenodactylin and other type 1 and type 2 RIPs (both toxic and non-toxic), phylogenetic trees were constructed based on the amino acid sequences of the A and the B chains of 11 families (Passifloraceae, Euphorbiaceae, Olacaceae, Theaceae, Lauraceae, Iridaceae, Santalaceae, Cucurbitaceae, Fabaceae, Asparagaceae and Adoxaceae) (Figure 8). The B-chain phylogenetic tree proved to be more reliable, with higher bootstrapping values for most of the branches. In this phylogenetic tree, proteins are segregated into two major clusters. One of them contains the non-toxic RIPs from the genera *Sambucus*, *Polygonatum*, *Momordica* and *Trichosanthes*; the other contains the toxic RIPs (including ricin and stenodactylin) but also non-toxic RIPs from the genera *Jatropha*, *Camellia*, *Cinnamomum*, *Iris* and *Trichosanthes*. Although the A-chain phylogenetic tree displays lower bootstrapping values (especially in the toxic RIP branch), it mostly reflects the B-chain tree. These phylogenetic trees suggest that toxic RIPs, such as stenodactylin or ricin, may appear in the evolution from a branch of non-toxic RIPs.

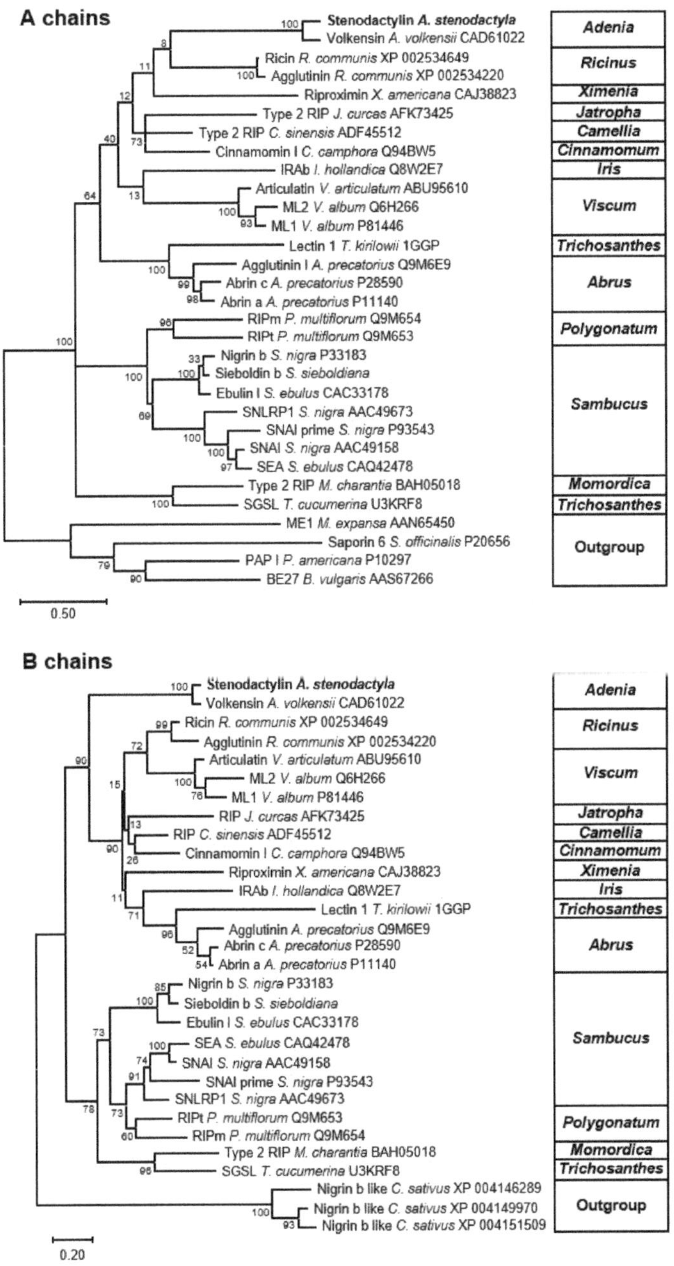

Figure 8. Molecular phylogenetic analysis by the Maximum Likelihood method of representative A and B-chain type 2 RIPs. The evolutionary history was inferred as indicated in the "Materials and Methods" section. The sequences of representative type 1 RIPs and monomeric lectins were used as the outgroup for the A and B chains, respectively. The name of the RIP (if any), the species and the accession number are indicated. All the sequences were retrieved and processed as indicated in the "Materials and Methods" section.

3. Discussion

In this paper, the complete amino acid sequence of stenodactylin was determined. Moreover, analysis of homology between stenodactylin and other RIPs was evaluated.

Sequence analysis showed that stenodactylin A and B chains contain 251 and 258 amino acids, respectively, corresponding to calculated Mr of about 28 kDa for both chains. The sugar presence could explain the difference between the molecular weight of the B chain based on the amino acid sequence (28 kDa) and the molecular weight observed by electrophoretic mobility (32 kDa) [7]. As reported for other type 2 RIPs, the A chain of stenodactylin contains only two lysines. Lysine residues are potential ubiquitination sites, and the small number of lysines is important to avoid ubiquitination and subsequent degradation [27]. In type 2 RIPs, the A and B chains are linked by a disulfide bridge between two cysteines. In ricin, the two cysteines that are involved are Cys259 of the A chain and Cys4 of the B chain [28]. Similarly, in stenodactylin Cys246 of A chain forms the disulfide bridge with Cys4 of B chain.

Based on the ricin A chain sequence, the key residues of active site are Tyr80, Tyr123, Glu177, Arg180 and Trp211 [15,29]. Near the active site, six other amino acids are important and conserved in both mono and bi-chain RIPs. These residues (Asn78, Arg134, Gln173, Ala178, Glu208 in ricin) are not directly involved in the depurination mechanism, but they help maintain the catalytic conformation [28,30]. The same amino acids of the active site are also conserved in the stenodactylin A chain (Tyr74, Tyr113, Glu163, Arg166, and Trp200).

As reported in the Introduction section, ricin B chain folds into two globular domains, each of which is composed of three subdomains. Only 1α and 2γ subdomains are involved in the galactose binding. The amino acids involved in the binding of galactose in the 1α site of ricin are Asp22, Asp25, Gln35 and Trp37, while the ones constituting the 2γ binding site are Asp234, Val235, Ala237, Tyr248 and His251 (Figure 6) [31]. Analysis of stenodactylin showed that all the amino acids that are involved in the first binding site of ricin are fully conserved (Asp22, Asp25, Gln35 and Trp37). In the 2γ binding site of stenodactylin, two amino acids are changed, compared to ricin; Ala237 and Tyr248 are replaced with Glu235 and His246 in stenodactylin, respectively. The substitution of Tyr by His was observed in volkensin [32], *R. communis* agglutinin [33] and *P. multiflorum* RIP [34]. Site-directed mutagenesis studies on the ricin B chain demonstrated that the replacement of Tyr248 with His248 reduced its binding activity [35]. The presence of a positive charge within the 2γ binding site prevents the hydrophobic interaction between the pyranose ring of galactose and the aromatic ring of Tyr; this substitution reduced functionality [34]. Cinnamomin contains three substitutions in the 2γ binding site compared with ricin (Gly239 for Ala237, Trp250 for Tyr248 and Thr253 for His251) (Figure 6). While the first substitution was conserved and the second one was between two aromatic amino acids, the third one removes a positive charge. As the lectin activity requires strictly conserved amino acids in both the 1α and 2γ domains, their change may explain the reduced cytotoxicity of cinnamonin [36]. Consistently, Tyr248 in ricin is replaced with Phe249 in ebulin l. These changes reduce the affinity of ebulin l for galactose-containing glycoproteins or glycolipids of the plasma membrane surface, thus reducing the cytotoxicity of the molecule [37,38]. On the other hand, non-toxic type 2 RIPs that are specific for sugars other than galactose have been reported. Thus, the tetrameric type 2 RIPs from species of the genus *Sambucus* (SNAI, SEA and SSA) are specific for Neu5Ac/galactose [39] and *Iris x hollandica* type 2 RIPs are specific for galactose/mannose [30]. In the case of the tetrameric RIPs from *Sambucus*, only the 2γ site is functional, because the 1α site has an additional cysteine involved in the linking between the two B-chains of the tetramer. Changes in the binding amino acids of the 2γ site, Glu235 by Gln, His246 by Tyr and His249 by Thr or Asn (Figure S3), allow the binding of galactose but also sialic acid [39]. In the type 2 RIPs from *Iris x hollandica* (IRAb and IRAr), changes occur in both 1α and 2γ sites, e.g., Trp37 by Ser and His246 by Trp (Figure S3), which allow the binding of both galactose and mannose [30].

All these data suggest that the 2γ binding site is important for the toxicity of RIPs, and any changes in this site could affect RIP binding. However, this hypothesis does not correlate with the results obtained with stenodactylin. In fact, stenodactylin, despite a change in this subdomain, is one of the most toxic RIPs.

According to the data reported in the literature [40], a high degree of identity was detected when the B chain of stenodactylin was compared with other B chains (90.3% with volkensin and ranging from 42.1 to 47.7% with the other RIPs). These data support the hypothesis that the B chain is a product of a gene duplication event [41]. The comparison of the stenodactylin A chain sequence with type 1 RIPs showed a very low level of identity. As above reported, the stenodactylin A chain showed a low degree of identity when compared with other type 2 RIP A chains, except for volkensin. Moreover, the identity of the A chains was lower than the identity of the B chains. The homology between the type 1 RIPs and the stenodactylin A chain was even lower than the identity calculated between the stenodactylin A chain and other type 2 RIP A chains.

The high cytotoxic potential of stenodactylin together with its ability to elicit in cancer cells a rapid stress response, leading mainly to apoptosis, but also triggering other cell death pathways, makes stenodactylin an ideal candidate as a pharmacological molecule for drug targeting in the experimental treatment of several cancer diseases. Due to its high systemic toxicity, native stenodactylin could only be employed for loco-regional treatments in cancer therapy. However, stenodactylin A-chain linked to a specific carrier by chemical conjugation or by genetic engineering, could find application to specifically target tumor cells in systemic therapy [11]. Moreover, stenodactylin may have an application in neurobiology. In fact, its characteristic retrograde transport in the peripheral nerves and central nervous system and its ability to kill neurons through different death pathways could be exploited to develop new molecular tools for experimental models of neurodegenerative diseases [9,10].

The knowledge of the stenodactylin sequence and structure may help to identify the amino acids directly or indirectly involved in RIP toxicity, thus stimulating research about this protein.

4. Materials and Methods

4.1. Materials

Stenodactylin was purified from the caudex of *Adenia stenodactyla* as described by Stripe and co-workers [7]. Adenia plants were purchased from Exotica Botanical Rarities (Erkelenz-golkrath, Germany) and, if not used immediately on arrival, were kept in the greenhouse of the Botanical Garden of the University of Bologna.

For RT-PCR analysis, the GenElute Mammalian Total RNA Kit and the primers were purchased from Sigma-Aldrich (St. Louis, MO, USA). For stenodactylin sequence the total RNA was isolated using the RNeasy Minikit, whereas the plasmids were purified by QIAfilter plasmid purification kit, both purchased from Qiagen (Hilden, Germany). The PCR products were purified using the High Pure PCR Product Purification kit obtained from Roche Applied Science (Penzberg, Germany). The reverse transcriptase MuLV, the dNTPs were obtained from GeneAmp RNA PCR kit (Roche). The chemically competent *E. coli* INVαF′ and the pCR®II cloning vectors were purchased from Invitrogen (Carlsbad, CA, USA).

The iScript cDNA synthesis Kit and the SsoFast™ EvaGreen® Supermix were obtained from Bio-Rad (Hercules, CA, USA). Other reagents used were from Merck (Darmstadt, Germany), Carlo Erba (Milano, Italy) and from Sigma.

Protein concentration was determined by UVICON 860 Spectrophotometer (Kontron Instruments, Milano, Italy). The DNA content was determined by a Beckman DU 640 spectrophotometer (Beckman, Brea, CA, USA). RT-PCR was performed using the CFX96 Real-Time PCR System (Bio-Rad).

PCR was conducted using the thermal cycler PCR system 2400 (Perkin Elmer, Waltham, MA, USA). Using DNA sequencing software, a search for sequence similarity was performed with the BLAST program available online [42]. The multiple sequence alignment program Clustal Omega [23] was used to detect the extent of sequence conservation and the secondary structure prediction was carried out using PSIPRED [22]. Glycosylation sites were predicted using the NetNGlyc1.0 server [19].

4.2. Methods

4.2.1. Synthesis of cDNA

The caudex of *A. stenodactyla* was disrupted using mortar and pestle and grinded to a fine powder under liquid nitrogen. Approximately 100 mg of total RNA was isolated using the RNeasy Minikit (Qiagen) according to the manufacturer's instruction. Poly(A)-rich RNA was reverse transcribed using the synthetic oligonucleotide T1 (5′ CGTCTAGAGTCGACTAGTGC(T)20 3′). Approximately 2 µg of total RNA and 1 µL of RNAse inhibitor were incubated at 65 °C in a thermal cycler for 5 min. It was later cooled on ice for 1 min and 15 µL of reaction mixture containing: 1 × PCR Buffer II, 5 mM of $MgCl_2$, 1 mM of each dNTP, 10 µM of T1, and 2.5 U/µL of MuLV reverse transcriptase (RNA PCR kit. Roche) was added. The reaction mixture was incubated for 20 min at 23 °C, then for 20 min at 42 °C, and finally 5 min at 99 °C.

The specific primers for the stenodactylin gene sequence were designed and synthesized based on the volkensin sequences (Table 2). Three pairs of primers were used to amplify the full-length cDNA sequence of stenodactylin: STA2-STB1R for A-chain; STA2-STB3R for A-chain and a piece of B-chain; STB1-STB5R for B-chain.

Table 2. Primer sequence.

Primer	Sequence
STA2	5′ GCCACGGTAGAGAGRTACACT 3′
STB1R	5′ AAGTCGTCTCCCCGGAAGGGC 3′
STB3R	5′ GGCGGGGTTGATGGTTCC 3′
STB1	5′ TGCCCTTCCGGGGAGACGACT 3′
STB5R	5′ TAGGAACCATTGCTGGTTGGA 3′

For cDNA amplification, 2 µL of the above-synthesize cDNA was used and 16 µL of master mix and 0.5 µM of each primer were added. A typical reaction master mix included: 1 × PCR buffer/Mg^{2+}, 0.25 mM dNTPs Mix, 2.5 U Taq Polymerase (Biotools, Madrid, Spain). PCR amplification was performed with the following conditions: an initial denaturation at 94 °C for 5 min, followed by 35 cycles of 94 °C for 30 s, 55–54 °C for 45 s and 72 °C for 2 min, and an additional extension of 10 min at 72 °C.

About 5 µL of amplified products from each tube was analyzed on 0.8% agarose gel.

As reported in Figure S1, the amplicons of expected size (about 0.85 kb for the A and B chains alone and about 1.1 kb for the combined A and small segment of B chains) were obtained, and the PCR products were purified using the High Pure PCR product Purification Kit (Roche) according to the manufacturer's instruction.

4.2.2. cDNA Cloning and Sequence

The three purified PCR fragments were ligated into the pCR®II vector and then were used to transform the Chemically Competent *E. coli* INVαF′ (Invitrogen) according to the manufacturer's instructions. Two clones for each fragment were purified and sequenced using M13 primers. DNA sequencing was carried out on the CENIT Support system (Villamayor-Salamnca, Spain).

4.2.3. Sequence Retrieval and Data Treatment

All the amino acid sequences of ribosome-inactivating proteins and lectins used in this study are available in the National Center for Biotechnology Information (NCBI) sequence database (https://www.ncbi.nlm.nih.gov/protein/), except those from sieboldin and SSA from *Sambucus sieboldiana* (Miq.) Blume ex Graebn., which were obtained from [43,44], respectively. For the representation logo and phylogenetic analysis, the signal peptide, and connecting peptide were removed using the following criteria by order of preference: information in the data bank entry, information in the literature from N-terminal sequencing, comparison with other close related sequences, and the use of the SignalP-5.0 Server (http://www.cbs.dtu.dk/services/SignalP/) [45].

4.2.4. Secondary Structure Prediction

The secondary structure was predicted using the PSIPRED Protein Structure Prediction Server (http://bioinf.cs.ucl.ac.uk/psipred/) [22].

4.2.5. Sequence Alignment

Sequence alignment was performed using the ClustalW tool included in the Mega X suite (https://www.megasoftware.net/) [23] with default parameters and edited manually to align the amino acids Tyr, Tyr, Glu, Arg, Trp in the active site of the A-chains, and all the Cys in the B-chains. Then, the sequences included between each pair of conserved amino acids were aligned automatically, and finally the complete sequences as well. Multiple sequence alignments were graphically represented by sequence logos [46] created with WebLogo 3 (http://weblogo.threeplusone.com/) [47]. The logos were created by using the A and B-chain sequences from 46 representative type 2 RIPs belonging to 28 plant species and limited to three, the maximum number of sequences for each species. For the representation of Figures 3, 4 and 6, the alignment was carried out using the Clustal Omega server (https://www.ebi.ac.uk/Tools/msa/clustalo/) [48].

4.2.6. Protein Structure Studies and Graphical Representation

The structure of ricin (accession number 2AAI) is available in the Protein Data Bank (https://www.rcsb.org/). Three-dimensional structural modelling of stenodactylin was carried out on the I-TASSER server (https://zhanglab.ccmb.med.umich.edu/I-TASSER/) [49]. Study and graph representations of protein structures were performed with the aid of the Discovery Studio Visualizer suite (v16.1.0) (https://www.3dsbiovia.com/).

4.2.7. Phylogenetic Analysis

The evolutionary histories of the A and B chains were inferred by using the Maximum Likelihood method and either the Whelan and Goldman [50] (for the A chain) or the JTT matrix-based [51] (for the B chain) models. The trees with the highest log likelihood (−13,115.61 for the A chain and −10,193.09 for the B chain) are shown. The percentage of trees in which the associated taxa clustered together is shown next to the branches. Initial trees for the heuristic search were obtained automatically by applying Neighbor-Join and BioNJ algorithms to a matrix of pairwise distances estimated using the JTT model, and then selecting the topology with superior log likelihood value. A discrete Gamma distribution was used to model evolutionary rate differences among sites (two categories (+G, parameter = 1.9285 for the A chain and 1.1766 for the B chain)). In the case of the A chain, the rate variation model allowed for some sites to be evolutionarily invariable (+I, 1.01% sites). The trees are drawn to scale, with branch lengths measured in the number of substitutions per site. This analysis involved 31 and 30 amino acid sequences for the A and B chains, respectively. There was a total of 346 and 314 positions in the final dataset for the A and B chains, respectively. Evolutionary analyses were conducted in MEGA X [23].

Supplementary Materials: The following are available online at http://www.mdpi.com/2072-6651/12/9/538/s1, Figure S1: Isolation of stenodactylin amplicons, Figure S2: Superimposition of stenodactylin and ricin structures, Figure S3: Alignment between the sugar-binding subdomains of stenodactylin, volkensin, ricin, abrin-a, SNAI, SSA, SEA, IRAb and IRAr.

Author Contributions: Conceptualization, R.I., A.B. and L.P.; methodology and validation, R.I. and J.M.F.; formal analysis and investigation, M.B., M.P. and L.C.; all the authors participated to write, review and edit the manuscript; funding acquisition, A.B., L.P. and J.M.F. All authors have read and agreed to the published version of the manuscript.

Funding: This work was supported by funds for selected research topics from the Alma Mater Studiorum, University of Bologna and by the Pallotti Legacies for Cancer Research; Fondazione CARISBO, Project 2019.0539; Grant VA033G19 (Consejería de Educación, Junta de Castilla y León) to the GIR ProtIBio.

Conflicts of Interest: The authors declare no conflict of interest.

References

1. Bolognesi, A.; Bortolotti, M.; Maiello, S.; Battelli, M.G.; Polito, L. Ribosome-Inactivating Proteins from Plants: A Historical Overview. *Molecules* **2016**, *21*, 1627. [CrossRef] [PubMed]
2. Polito, L.; Bortolotti, M.; Maiello, S.; Battelli, M.G.; Bolognesi, A. Plants Producing Ribosome-Inactivating Proteins in Traditional Medicine. *Molecules* **2016**, *21*, 1560. [CrossRef] [PubMed]
3. Bortolotti, M.; Mercatelli, D.; Polito, L. *Momordica charantia*, a Nutraceutical Approach for Inflammatory Related Diseases. *Front. Pharmacol.* **2019**, *10*, 486. [CrossRef] [PubMed]
4. Barbieri, L.; Valbonesi, P.; Bonora, E.; Gorini, P.; Bolognesi, A.; Stirpe, F. Polynucleotide:adenosine glycosidase activity of ribosome-inactivating proteins: Effect on DNA, RNA and poly(A). *Nucleic Acids Res.* **1997**, *25*, 518–522. [CrossRef] [PubMed]
5. Battelli, M.G.; Barbieri, L.; Bolognesi, A.; Buonamici, L.; Valbonesi, P.; Polito, L.; Van Damme, E.J.M.; Peumans, W.J.; Stirpe, F. Ribosome-inactivating lectins with polynucleotide:adenosine glycosidase activity. *FEBS Lett.* **1997**, *408*, 355–359. [CrossRef]
6. Polito, L.; Bortolotti, M.; Battelli, M.G.; Calafato, G.; Bolognesi, A. Ricin: An Ancient Story for a Timeless Plant Toxin. *Toxins* **2019**, *11*, 324. [CrossRef]
7. Stirpe, F.; Bolognesi, A.; Bortolotti, M.; Farini, V.; Lubelli, C.; Pelosi, E.; Polito, L.; Dozza, B.; Strocchi, P.; Chambery, A.; et al. Characterization of highly toxic type 2 ribosome-inactivating proteins from *Adenia lanceolata* and *Adenia stenodactyla* (Passifloraceae). *Toxicon* **2007**, *50*, 94–105. [CrossRef]
8. Wiley, R.G.; Kline, R.H., IV. Neuronal lesioning with axonally transported toxins. *J. Neurosci. Methods* **2000**, *103*, 73–82. [CrossRef]
9. Monti, B.; D'Alessandro, C.; Farini, V.; Bolognesi, A.; Polazzi, E.; Contestabile, A.; Stirpe, F.; Battelli, M.G. In vitro and in vivo toxicity of type 2 ribosome-inactivating proteins lanceolin and stenodactylin on glial and neuronal cells. *Neurotoxicology* **2007**, *28*, 637–644. [CrossRef]
10. Polito, L.; Bortolotti, M.; Pedrazzi, M.; Mercatelli, D.; Battelli, M.G.; Bolognesi, A. Apoptosis and necroptosis induced by stenodactylin in neuroblastoma cells can be completely prevented through caspase inhibition plus catalase or necrostatin-1. *Phytomedicine* **2016**, *23*, 32–41. [CrossRef]
11. Mercatelli, D.; Bortolotti, M.; Andresen, V.; Sulen, A.; Polito, L.; Gjertsen, B.T.; Bolognesi, A. Early response to the plant toxin stenodactylin in acute myeloid leukemia cells involves inflammatory and apoptotic signaling. *Front. Pharmacol.* **2020**, *11*, 630. [CrossRef] [PubMed]
12. Polito, L.; Djemil, A.; Bortolotti, M. Plant Toxin-Based Immunotoxins for Cancer Therapy: A Short Overview. *Biomedicines* **2016**, *4*, 12. [CrossRef] [PubMed]
13. Puri, M.; Kaur, I.; Perugini, M.A.; Gupta, R.C. Ribosome-inactivating proteins: Current status and biomedical applications. *Drug Discov. Today* **2012**, *17*, 774–783. [CrossRef] [PubMed]
14. De Virgilio, M.; Lombardi, A.; Caliandro, R.; Fabbrini, M.S. Ribosome-inactivating proteins: From plant defense to tumor attack. *Toxins* **2010**, *2*, 2699–2737. [CrossRef]
15. Montfort, W.; Villafranca, J.E.; Monzingo, A.F.; Ernst, S.R.; Katzin, B.; Rutenber, E.; Xuong, N.H.; Hamlin, R.; Robertus, J.D. The three-dimensional structure of ricin at 2.8 A. *J. Biol. Chem.* **1987**, *262*, 5398–5403.
16. Mlsna, D.; Monzingo, A.F.; Katzin, B.J.; Ernst, S.; Robertus, J.D. Structure of recombinant ricin A chain at 2.3 A. *Protein Sci.* **1993**, *2*, 429–435. [CrossRef]
17. Tosi, G.; Fermani, S.; Falini, G.; Polito, L.; Bortolotti, M.; Bolognesi, A. Crystallization and preliminary X-ray diffraction data analysis of stenodactylin, a highly toxic type 2 ribosome-inactivating protein from *Adenia stenodactyla*. *Acta Crystallogr. Sect. F Struct. Biol. Cryst. Commun.* **2010**, *66*, 51–53. [CrossRef]
18. ExPASy Bioinformatics Resource Portal. Available online: https://www.expasy.org/ (accessed on 25 June 2020).
19. NetNGlyc 1.0 Server. Available online: http://www.cbs.dtu.dk/services/NetNGlyc/ (accessed on 25 June 2020).
20. Yan, Q.; Li, X.P.; Tumer, N.E. N-glycosylation does not affect the catalytic activity of ricin A chain but stimulates cytotoxicity by promoting its transport out of the endoplasmic reticulum. *Traffic* **2012**, *13*, 1508–1521. [CrossRef]

21. Sehgal, P.; Kumar, O.; Kameswararao, M.; Ravindran, J.; Khan, M.; Sharma, S.; Vijayaraghavan, R.; Prasad, G.B.K.S. Differential toxicity profile of ricin isoforms correlates with their glycosylation levels. *Toxicology* **2011**, *282*, 56–67. [CrossRef]
22. Buchan, D.W.A.; Jones, D.T. The PSIPRED Protein Analysis Workbench: 20 years on. *Nucleic Acids Res.* **2019**, *47*, W402–W407. [CrossRef]
23. Kumar, S.; Stecher, G.; Li, M.; Knyaz, C.; Tamura, K. MEGA X: Molecular Evolutionary Genetics Analysis across Computing Platforms. *Mol. Biol. Evol.* **2018**, *35*, 1547–1549. [CrossRef] [PubMed]
24. Rutenber, E.; Katzin, B.J.; Ernst, S.; Collins, E.J.; Mlsna, D.; Ready, M.P.; Robertus, J.D. Crystallographic refinement of ricin to 2.5 A. *Proteins* **1991**, *10*, 240–250. [CrossRef] [PubMed]
25. Tahirov, T.H.; Lu, T.H.; Liaw, Y.C.; Chen, Y.L.; Lin, J.Y. Crystal structure of abrin-a at 2.14 A. *J. Mol. Biol.* **1995**, *250*, 354–367. [CrossRef] [PubMed]
26. Di Maro, A.; Citores, L.; Russo, R.; Iglesias, R.; Ferreras, J.M. Sequence comparison and phylogenetic analysis by the Maximum Likelihood method of ribosome-inactivating proteins from angiosperms. *Plant Mol. Biol.* **2014**, *85*, 575–588. [CrossRef]
27. Deeks, E.D.; Cook, J.P.; Day, P.J.; Smith, D.C.; Roberts, L.M.; Lord, J.M. The low lysine content of ricin a chain reduces the risk of proteolytic degradation after translocation from the endoplasmic reticulum to the cytosol. *Biochemistry* **2002**, *41*, 3405–3413. [CrossRef]
28. Katzin, B.J.; Collins, E.J.; Robertus, J.D. Structure of ricin A-chain at 2.5 A. *Proteins* **1991**, *10*, 251–259. [CrossRef]
29. Monzingo, A.F.; Robertus, J.D. X-ray analysis of substrate analogs in the ricin A-chain active site. *J. Mol. Biol.* **1992**, *227*, 1136–1145. [CrossRef]
30. Hao, Q.; Van Damme, E.J.; Hause, B.; Barre, A.; Chen, Y.; Rougé, P.; Peumans, W.J. Iris bulbs express type 1 and type 2 ribosome-inactivating proteins with unusual properties. *Plant Physiol.* **2001**, *125*, 866–876. [CrossRef]
31. Rutenber, E.; Robertus, J.D. Structure of ricin B-chain at 2.5 A resolution. *Proteins* **1991**, *10*, 260–269. [CrossRef]
32. Chambery, A.; Di Maro, A.; Monti, M.M.; Stirpe, F.; Parente, A. Volkensin from Adenia volkensii Harms (kilyambiti plant), a type 2 ribosome-inactivating protein. *Eur. J. Biochem.* **2004**, *271*, 108–117. [CrossRef]
33. Roberts, L.M.; Lamb, F.I.; Pappin, D.J.; Lord, J.M. The primary sequence of *Ricinus communis* agglutinin. Comparison with ricin. *J. Biol. Chem.* **1985**, *260*, 15682–15686. [PubMed]
34. Van Damme, E.J.; Hao, Q.; Charels, D.; Barre, A.; Rougé, P.; Van Leuven, F.; Peumans, W.J. Characterization and molecular cloning of two different type 2 ribosome-inactivating proteins from the monocotyledonous plant *Polygonatum multiflorum*. *Eur. J. Biochem.* **2000**, *267*, 2746–2759. [CrossRef] [PubMed]
35. Lehar, S.M.; Pedersen, J.T.; Kamath, R.S.; Swimmer, C.; Goldmacher, V.S.; Lambert, J.M.; Blättler, W.A.; Guild, B.C. Mutational and structural analysis of the lectin activity in binding domain 2 of ricin B chain. *Protein Eng.* **1994**, *7*, 1261–1266. [CrossRef] [PubMed]
36. Wang, B.Z.; Zou, W.G.; Liu, W.Y.; Liu, X.Y. The lower cytotoxicity of cinnamomin (a type II RIP) is due to its B-chain. *Arch. Biochem. Biophys.* **2006**, *451*, 91–96. [CrossRef] [PubMed]
37. Pascal, J.M.; Day, P.J.; Monzingo, A.F.; Ernst, S.R.; Robertus, J.D.; Iglesias, R.; Pérez, Y.; Ferreras, J.M.; Citores, L.; Girbés, T. 2.8-A crystal structure of a nontoxic type-II ribosome-inactivating protein, ebulin l. *Proteins* **2001**, *43*, 319–326. [CrossRef] [PubMed]
38. Ferreras, J.M.; Citores, L.; Iglesias, R.; Jiménez, P.; Girbés, T. Sambucus Ribosome-Inactivating Proteins and Lectins. Toxic Plant Proteins. In *Toxic Plant Proteins–Plant Cell Monographs*, 1st ed.; Lord, J.M., Hartley, M.R., Eds.; Springer: Berlin/Heidelberg, Germany, 2010; Volume 18, pp. 107–131. [CrossRef]
39. Iglesias, R.; Ferreras, J.M.; Di Maro, A.; Citores, L. Ebulin-RP, a novel member of the Ebulin gene family with low cytotoxicity as a result of deficient sugar binding domains. *Biochim. Biophys. Acta Gen. Subj.* **2018**, *1862*, 460–473. [CrossRef]
40. Barbieri, L.; Battelli, M.G.; Stirpe, F. Ribosome-inactivating proteins from plants. *Biochim. Biophys. Acta.* **1993**, *1154*, 237–282. [CrossRef]
41. Villafranca, J.E.; Robertus, J.D. Ricin B chain is a product of gene duplication. *J. Biol. Chem.* **1981**, *256*, 554–556.
42. Blast-Basic Local Alignment Search Tool. Available online: https://blast.ncbi.nlm.nih.gov/Blast.cgi (accessed on 25 June 2020).

43. Rojo, M.A.; Yato, M.; Ishii-Minami, N.; Minami, E.; Kaku, H.; Citores, L.; Girbés, T.; Shibuya, N. Isolation, cDNA cloning, biological properties, and carbohydrate binding specificity of sieboldin-b, a type II ribosome-inactivating protein from the bark of japanese elderberry (*Sambucus sieboldiana*). *Arch. Biochem. Biophys.* **1997**, *340*, 185–194. [CrossRef]
44. Kaku, H.; Tanaka, Y.; Tazaki, K.; Minami, E.; Mizuno, H.; Shibuya, N. Sialylated oligosaccharide-specific plant lectin from japanese elderberry (*Sambucus sieboldiana*) bark tissue has a homologous structure to type II ribosome-inactivating proteins, ricin and abrin: CDNA cloning and molecular modeling study. *J. Biol. Chem.* **1996**, *271*, 1480–1485. [CrossRef]
45. Almagro Armenteros, J.J.; Tsirigos, K.D.; Sønderby, C.K.; Nordahl Petersen, T.; Winther, O.; Brunak, S.; von Heijne, G.; Nielsen, H. SignalP 5.0 improves signal peptide predictions using deep neural networks. *Nat. Biotechnol.* **2019**, *37*, 420–423. [CrossRef] [PubMed]
46. Schneider, T.D.; Stephens, R.M. Sequence logos: A new way to display consensus sequences. *Nucleic Acids Res.* **1990**, *18*, 6097–6100. [CrossRef] [PubMed]
47. Crooks, G.E.; Hon, G.; Chandonia, J.M.; Brenner, S.E. WebLogo: A sequence logo generator. *Genome Res.* **2004**, *14*, 1188–1190. [CrossRef] [PubMed]
48. Sievers, F.; Wilm, A.; Dineen, D.; Gibson, T.J.; Karplus, K.; Li, W.; Lopez, R.; McWilliam, H.; Remmert, M.; Söding, J.; et al. Fast, scalable generation of high-quality protein multiple sequence alignments using Clustal Omega. *Mol. Syst. Biol.* **2011**, *7*, 539. [CrossRef]
49. Yang, J.; Zhang, Y. I-TASSER server: New development for protein structure and function predictions. *Nucleic Acids Res.* **2015**, *43*, W174–W181. [CrossRef]
50. Whelan, S.; Goldman, N. A general empirical model of protein evolution derived from multiple protein families using a maximum-likelihood approach. *Mol. Biol. Evol.* **2001**, *18*, 691–699. [CrossRef]
51. Jones, D.T.; Taylor, W.R.; Thornton, J.M. The rapid generation of mutation data matrices from protein sequences. *Comput. Appl. Biosci.* **1992**, *8*, 275–282. [CrossRef]

toxins

MDPI

Article

Pseudomonas Exotoxin A Based Toxins Targeting Epidermal Growth Factor Receptor for the Treatment of Prostate Cancer

Alexandra Fischer [1,2], Isis Wolf [1,2], Hendrik Fuchs [3], Anie Priscilla Masilamani [1,2] and Philipp Wolf [1,2,*]

1 Faculty of Medicine, University of Freiburg, 79106 Freiburg, Germany; alexandra.fischer.uro@uniklinik-freiburg.de (A.F.); isis.wolf@uniklinik-freiburg.de (I.W.); anie.priscilla.masilamani@uniklinik-freiburg.de (A.P.M.)

2 Department of Urology, Antibody-Based Diagnostics and Therapies, Medical Center—University of Freiburg, Breisacher Str. 66, 79106 Freiburg, Germany

3 Institute of Laboratory Medicine, Clinical Chemistry and Pathobiochemistry, Charité—Universitätsmedizin Berlin, corporate member of Freie Universität Berlin, Humboldt-Universität zu Berlin, and Berlin Institute of Health, 13353 Berlin, Germany; hendrik.fuchs@charite.de

* Correspondence: philipp.wolf@uniklinik-freiburg.de; Tel.: +49-761-270-28921

Received: 30 September 2020; Accepted: 26 November 2020; Published: 28 November 2020

Abstract: The epidermal growth factor receptor (EGFR) was found to be a valuable target on prostate cancer (PCa) cells. However, EGFR inhibitors mostly failed in clinical studies with patients suffering from PCa. We therefore tested the targeted toxins EGF-PE40 and EGF-PE24mut consisting of the natural ligand EGF as binding domain and PE40, the natural toxin domain of *Pseudomonas* Exotoxin A, or PE24mut, the de-immunized variant thereof, as toxin domains. Both targeted toxins were expressed in the periplasm of *E.coli* and evoked an inhibition of protein biosynthesis in EGFR-expressing PCa cells. Concentration- and time-dependent killing of PCa cells was found with IC_{50} values after 48 and 72 h in the low nanomolar or picomolar range based on the induction of apoptosis. EGF-PE24mut was found to be about 11- to 120-fold less toxic than EGF-PE40. Both targeted toxins were more than 600 to 140,000-fold more cytotoxic than the EGFR inhibitor erlotinib. Due to their high and specific cytotoxicity, the EGF-based targeted toxins EGF-PE40 and EGF-PE24mut represent promising candidates for the future treatment of PCa.

Keywords: prostate cancer; targeted toxins; epidermal growth factor; epidermal growth factor receptor; *Pseudomonas* Exotoxin A

Key Contribution: We generated the first targeted toxins consisting of EGF as binding and the enzymatic active domain of *Pseudomonas aeruginosa* Exotoxin A as toxin domain. The immunotoxins showed high and specific cytotoxicity against EGFR expressing PCa cells and are promising candidates for a future therapy of PCa.

1. Introduction

Prostate cancer (PCa) is the second most common malignancy in men worldwide. More than 1.27 million new cases and more than 358,000 deaths are expected from this tumor every year [1]. Primary tumors can be successfully treated by surgery or local radiation. However, despite improved therapeutic options, such as androgen deprivation therapy, radiation, and chemotherapy, curative treatment is no longer possible, once the tumor has spread [2].

In recent years, targeted therapy has been established as a new cornerstone beside the classical treatment options for advanced PCa [3–5]. In the search for antigens that could serve as targets, the focus, among the prostate specific membrane antigen (PSMA) [5,6] or the prostate stem cell antigen (PSCA) [7], has been on the epidermal growth factor receptor (EGFR) [8–10]. EGFR belongs to the ErbB receptor tyrosine kinase family [11]. It is a 1186 amino acid transmembrane glycoprotein comprised of an *N*-terminal 621 amino acid (aa) extracellular domain, a 23 aa transmembrane domain, and a 542 aa cytoplasmic domain including tyrosine kinase activity and *C*-terminal phosphorylation sites [12,13]. Seven ligands were described to bind to EGFR: the epidermal growth factor (EGF), the transforming growth factor α (TGFα), amphiregulin, betacellulin, epigen, epiregulin, and the heparin binding EGF-like growth factor [14]. After ligand binding, EGFR homodimerizes or heterodimerizes with other members of the ErbB family (HER2/ErbB2, ErbB3, or ErbB4) followed by autophosphorylation of the intracellular tyrosine kinase domain and activation of signaling pathways associated with cell proliferation, growth, differentiation, migration, and apoptosis inhibition [15].

EGFR signaling was found to play a major role in the tumorigenesis of PCa in view of proliferation, survival, invasiveness, and metastasis [16–19]. In different studies, EGFR expression was found in 18–75.9% of patients with prostate adenocarcinoma and in 100% of patients with hormone-refractory metastatic disease [20–22]. EGFR overexpression was significantly associated with Gleason score, recurrence, castration resistant disease, and poorer disease-free survival [20–22]. Moreover, EGFR mediates docetaxel resistance in human castration-resistant PCa through the Akt-dependent expression of ABCB1 (MDR1) [23].

Different inhibitors against EGFR, like Erlotinib, Gefitinib, Vandetanib (which additionally inhibits VEGF), and Lapatinib (which additionally inhibits HER2) were tested alone or in combination with chemotherapy in phase II studies on patients with castration resistant PCa [24–27]. However, results were disappointing and no or only low anti-cancer activity in some patients could be registered. Treatment of patients with the anti-EGFR mAb Cetuximab plus Docetaxel were more promising. In 20% and 31% of the patients, a >50% and >30% decline, respectively, of the serum tumor marker prostate specific antigen (PSA) was reached with a significant improved progression-free survival in patients with EGFR overexpression [28].

EGFR can not only serve as a target for antibodies or inhibitors, which are intended to downregulate EGFR-dependent signaling pathways. Since EGFR is internalized into the cell after ligand or antibody binding [29,30], it can also be used as a carrier for the targeted delivery of toxins that unfold their cytotoxicity inside the cancer cells.

Various targeted toxins against EGFR were therefore generated in the past and tested against different hematological and solid tumors. The anti-EGFR mAbs cetuximab or panitumumab, anti-EGFR scFv thereof, TGFα, or EGF, were used as binding domains and enzymatic active domains of ribosome-inactivating proteins, like *Pseudomonas* Exotoxin A, Saporin, Dianthin, or Diphtheria toxin, were used as toxin domains (rev. in [31]). Yip and colleagues developed a conjugate consisting of the chimeric murine-human mAb cetuximab bound to Saporin by a biotin-streptavidin linker. Cytotoxicity against DU145 PCa cells was enhanced by photochemical internalization, leading to direct release of the conjugate from the endo-lysosomal compartment into the cytosol [32]. Targeted toxins consisting of the anti-EGFR scFv2112 from cetuximab or scFv1711 from panitumumab and the truncated version of *Pseudomonas* Exotoxin A (ETA′) were also tested against different tumor entities, including PCa. A high and specific cytotoxicity was determined on C4-2 PCa cells [29].

Due to the murine origin of their binding domains and the bacterial or plant origin of their toxin domains, targeted toxins are considered immunogenic in patients, which makes clinical use risky [33]. In the present study, we therefore generated new recombinant anti-EGFR targeted toxins for the treatment of PCa. We chose the natural human EGF ligand as binding domain and PE40, the *C*-terminal part of *Pseudomonas* Exotoxin A (PE), lacking the CD91 binding domain I and consisting of the domains II, Ib, and III with 40 kDa in size, as the toxin domain. Moreover, we generated a targeted toxin variant with EGF and a de-immunized PE domain, called PE24mut. In this toxic domain of 24 kDa in size, parts of domain II containing immunodominant B- and T-cell epitopes are deleted and only the furin cleavage site is retained. Moreover, seven immunodominant B-cell epitopes of domain III are mutated to alanines (R427A, R458A, D463A, R467A, R490A, R505A, R538A) [34]. We tested the targeted toxins EFG-PE40 and EGF-PE24mut on different PCa cell lines, representing advanced stages of the disease, in view of protein biosynthesis inhibition, cytotoxicity and induction of apoptosis. We found that both are promising candidates for further development to be used for the future treatment of PCa.

2. Results

2.1. Cloning, Expression and Purification of EGF and the Targeted Toxins EGF-PE40 and EGF-PE24mut

The natural EGF ligand and the targeted toxins EGF-PE40 and EGF-PE24mut were generated by cloning EGF via *NcoI/NotI* restriction sites into the vector pHOG21 containing a c-myc and a His-tag for detection and purification, followed by the insertion of the PE40 or PE24mut domains via *XbaI* restriction site (Figure 1).

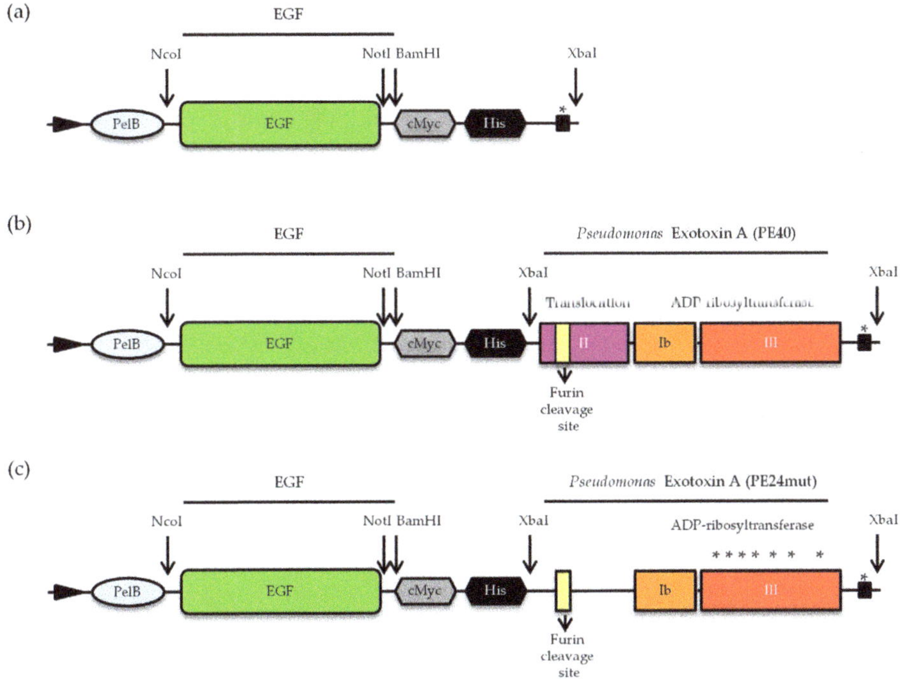

Figure 1. Cloning of EGF and the targeted toxins EGF-PE40 and EGF-PE24mut. Schematic representation of (**a**) EGF, (**b**), EGF-PE40, and (**c**) EFG-PE24mut in the vector pHOG21. (Abbreviations: *c-myc*, human c-myc tag; *His*$_6$, hexahistidine tag; *PelB*, pel B leader for periplasmatic expression. * Mutations of amino acids within immunodominant epitopes to alanine for de-immunization.

For expression and purification, vector DNA of EGF, EGF-PE40 and EGF-PE24mut was transformed into *E.coli* XL-1 blue bacteria and purified via immobilized metal affinity chromatography (IMAC) with a purity yield of approx. 95%, 82%, and 82%, respectively, as quantified by densiometric quantification of the SDS gels (Figure 2a,c,e). Western Blot analysis using anti c-myc antibody clearly identified the expression of the three proteins that appeared at their expected molecular masses in elution fractions, namely EGF at 8.4 kDa, EGF-PE40 at 49.2 kDa and EGF-PE24mut at 34.7 kDa (Figure 2b,d,f).

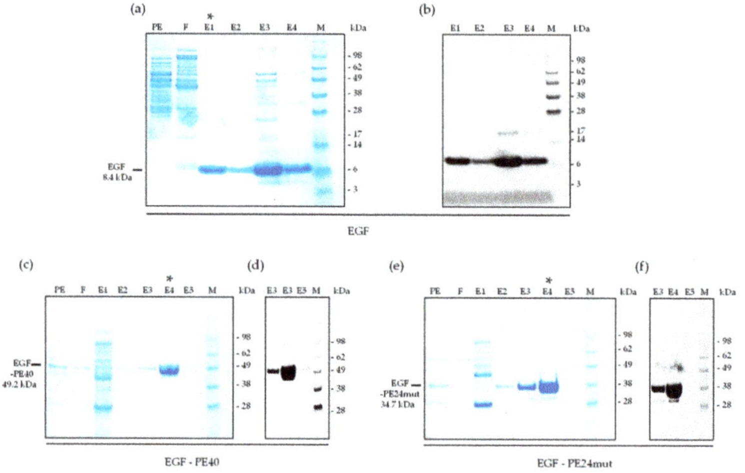

Figure 2. Expression and purification of EGF, EGF-PE40, and EGF-PE24mut. (**a**) SDS-PAGE and (**b**) Western Blot of purified EGF found in the elution fractions E1-E4. (**c**) SDS-PAGE and (**d**) Western Blot of purified EGF-PE40 found in the elution fractions E2-E4. (**e**) SDS-PAGE and (**f**) Western Blot of purified EGF-PE24mut found in the elution fractions E2-E4. * elution fraction with highest purity used for the following experiments. Abbreviations: E1–4, elution fractions 1–4; F, flow-through; M, marker; PE, periplasmatic extract.

2.2. Binding of EGF-PE40 and EGF-PE24mut to Different PCa Cell Lines

EGFR expression was evaluated on the PCa cell lines LNCaP, DU145, and PC-3 by Western Blot using anti-EGFR rabbit pAb (Figure 3a). Abundant EGFR expression was found in all three PCa lines after flow cytometric analysis with 98.6% of positive population in LNCaP, 99.7% of positive population in DU145 and 96.5% of positive population in PC-3 cells (Figure 3b).

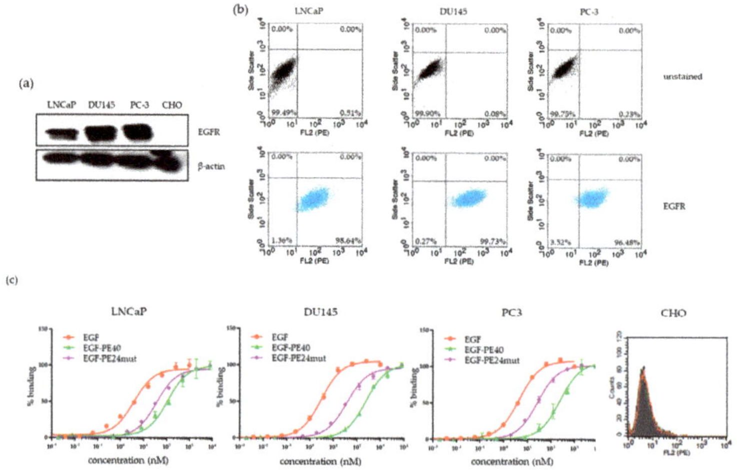

Figure 3. EGFR expression and EGF binding to different PCa cell lines. (**a**) EGFR expression on different PCa cell lines (LNCaP, DU145, PC-3) and CHO control cells as shown by Western Blot. (**b**) Flow cytometric analysis of EGFR-positive cell populations in LNCaP, DU145, PC-3 and EGFR-negative CHO cells. (**c**) Binding of EGF, EGF-PE40, and EGF-PE24mut to PCa cells at saturated concentration on PSMA-negative CHO cells.

Equilibrium dissociation constants (K_D) of 3.8, 3.1, and 4.4 nM were determined for EGF on LNCaP, DU145, and PC-3 cells, respectively (Figure 3c, Table S1). Compared to EGF, binding of EGF-PE40 was 28.6- to 76.1-fold reduced and binding of EGF-PE24mut was 6.0- to 11.9-fold reduced. No binding at saturated concentrations was seen on PSMA-negative CHO control cells.

2.3. EGF-PE40 and EGF-PE24mut Inhibit Protein Biosynthesis

Since PE-based targeted toxins are known to inhibit the protein biosynthesis of target cells by ADP-ribosylation of eEF-2 [35], we checked whether there was an inhibition of protein biosynthesis in our cells lines after incubation with our constructs. Protein biosynthesis inhibition was analyzed using puromycin before lysis of the intoxicated cells. The antibiotic puromycin acts as an analog of the 3′aminoacyl-tRNA, causing the formation of puromycylated nascent chains [36,37]. The inhibition of protein biosynthesis can then be detected by Western Blotting using an anti-puromycin antibody. In all EGFR-positive PCa cell lines, a stronger protein biosynthesis inhibition with EGF-PE40 compared to EGF-PE24mut was found. Whereas EGF-PE40 led to nearly complete inhibition of protein biosynthesis after the mentioned time intervals in all PCa cell lines, EGF-PE24mut showed only partial protein biosynthesis inhibition in DU145 and PC-3 cells. No inhibition was observed in EGFR-negative CHO cells (Figure 4).

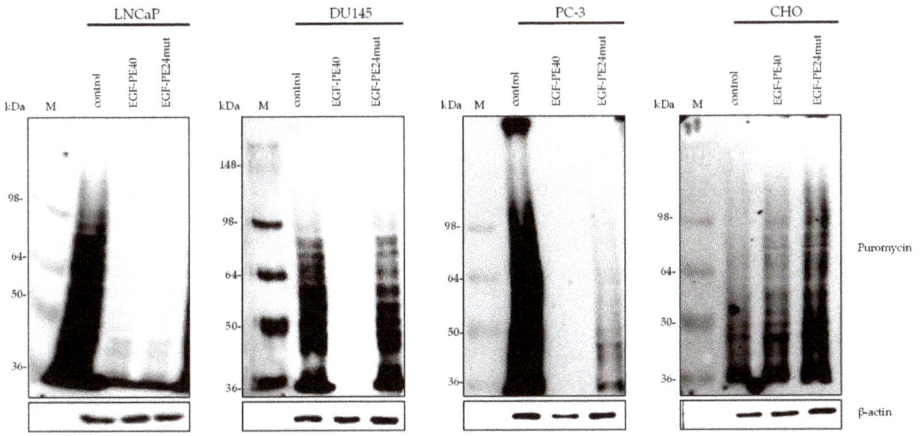

Figure 4. Protein biosynthesis inhibition in PCa as shown by puromycin Western Blot. EGF-PE40 and EGF-PE24mut inhibited protein biosynthesis of LNCaP cells after 48 h incubation with 0.7 nM EGF-PE40 or EGF-PE24mut, of DU145 cells after 72 h incubation with 1 nM of the targeted toxins, and of PC-3 as well as CHO cells after 72 h incubation with 2 nM of the targeted toxins.

2.4. EGF-PE40 and EGF-PE24mut Reduce Cell Viability and Induce Apoptosis

Upon treatment of the PCa cells with EGF-PE40 or EGF-PE24mut, explicit morphological changes were observed in the PCa cells pointing towards cell death, whereas no signs of cell death or morphological changes were observed in CHO cells (Figure S1). Using WST-1 viability assay, we found that EGF-PE40 and EGF-PE24mut specifically reduced the viability of all PCa cell lines in a time and concentration dependent manner (Figure 5a, Table 1).

With EGF-PE40, IC_{50} values of 0.008 nM, 0.18 nM, and 0.86 nM were calculated for LNCaP, DU145, and PC-3 cells after 72 h incubation, respectively. For EGF-PE24mut, IC_{50} values of 0.97 nM, 5.27 nM, and 9.59 nM could be determined at the same time. Thus, they were about 11- to 120-fold lower compared to the IC_{50} values of EGF-PE40. No reduction in cell viability was observed in EGFR-negative CHO cells (Figure 5a, Table 1).

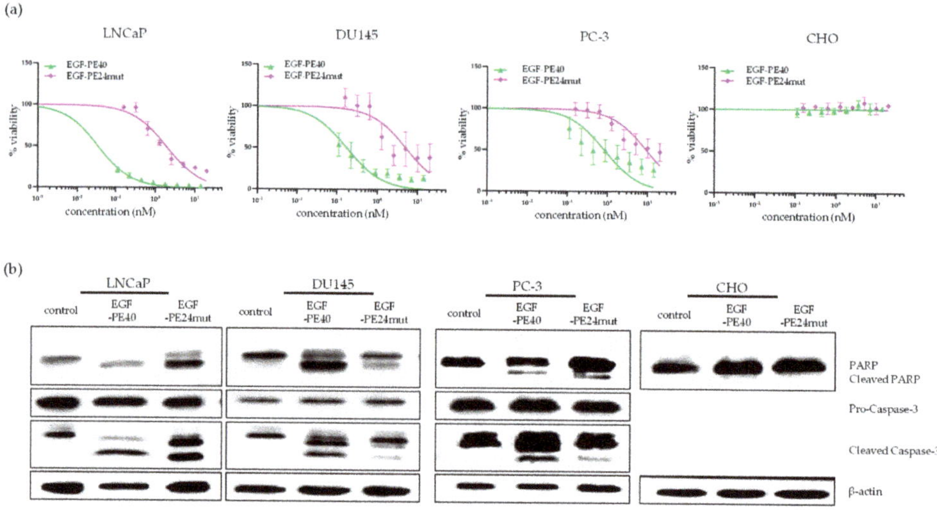

Figure 5. EGF targeted toxins reduce cell viability and induce apoptosis. (**a**) EGFR-positive LNCaP, DU145, PC-3 and EGFR-negative CHO cells were incubated with EGF-PE40 or EGF-PE24mut for 48 (LNCaP) or 72 h (DU145, PC-3 and CHO cells), respectively. Reduction of cell viability was calculated by WST-1 assay. Mean values ± SEM of three independent experiments. (**b**) Western Blots of the apoptotic markers PARP, cleaved PARP, Caspase-3 and cleaved Caspase-3 after incubation of the cells with EGF-PE40 or EGF-PE24mut at the same time points. β-actin was used as loading control.

Table 1. IC_{50} values of EGF-PE40, EGF-PE24mut, and erlotinib on PCa cells. CHO cells served as control. IC_{50} values, defined as half-maximal inhibitory concentrations, were determined using WST-1 viability assay and GraphPad Prism 7 software.

	LNCaP			**DU145**			**PC-3**			**CHO**		
	IC_{50}(nM)			**IC_{50}(nM)**			**IC_{50}(nM)**			**IC_{50}(nM)**		
	24h	48h	72h	24h	48h	72h	24h	48h	72h	24h	48h	72h
EGF-PE40	2.31	0.04	0.008	2.71	0.31	0.18	9.67	0.64	0.86	>14.5	>14.5	>14.5
EGF-PE24mut	>20.6	1.91	0.97	>20.6	8.52	5.27	>20.6	8.80	9.59	>20.6	>20.6	>20.6
Erlotinib	nd	>5750	nd	nd	nd	>5750	nd	nd	>5750	nd	nd	>5750

To evaluate the cause of cell death, PARP cleavage and Caspase-3 cleavage were checked as markers for apoptosis by Western Blot analysis. PARP and Caspase-3 cleavage were observed in LNCaP (48 h), DU145 (72 h) and PC-3 (72 h) cell lines after treatment with EGF-PE40 and EGF-PE24mut with tendency to a higher degree in EGF-PE40 treated cells. No PARP cleavage was observed in CHO cells (Figure 5b). In contrast to the EGF-targeted toxins, the EGFR inhibitor erlotinib showed no measurable cytotoxicity in the PCa cells up to a concentration of 5750 nM after 72 h (Table 1, Figure S2). Thus, EGF-PE40 was more than 6680 to 140,000-fold and EGF-PE24mut more than 600 to 3000-fold cytotoxic than erlotinib. Whole Western Blots including densitometry ratios are in Figure S3.

3. Discussion

We have successfully generated new targeted toxins that bind to EGFR and effectively induce apoptosis in androgen-dependent and independent growing PCa cells, which represent different stages of advanced disease [38].

Clinical studies with PE-based targeted toxins against various solid malignancies have shown formation of anti-drug antibodies (ADA) against the non-human binding domains and against the bacterial toxin domains leading to dangerous side effects and discontinuation of therapy [39]. The focus is therefore increasingly on the generation of targeted toxins with lower immunogenicity.

We used the natural ligand EGF as binding domain for our targeted toxins, which has the advantage over murine or chimeric anti-EGFR antibodies or scFv (scFv) [32,40] that it should not be immunogenic due to its human origin. As toxin domain, we used the naturally occurring cytotoxic domain of *Pseudomonas* Exotoxin A, PE40, and a de-immunized variant thereof, called PE24mut, which was shown to reduce the immunogenicity of the bacterial domain [34]. With the use of *Pseudomonas* Exotoxin A, we exploited the originally harmful properties of this virulence factor, which developed during evolution, for the therapy of cancer cells [41]. These properties include the formation of a furin cleavable motif within domain II for effective endosomal release of the toxin domain and a *N*-terminal KDEL-like motif for retrograde transport of the toxin domain via the Golgi apparatus to the ER. Furthermore, a translocation domain for passage through biological membranes has been formed as well as the ability to specifically ADP-ribosylate diphthamide, an amino acid that has so far only been described in eEF-2 [42].

We found that cell binding of EGF was reduced by addition of the PE24mut toxin domain and to an even greater extent by addition of the PE40 domain. It can thus be assumed that there was some steric inhibition of the EFG ligand by the toxin domains. The lower binding of EGF-PE40 compared to EGF-PE24mut, however, did not lead to reduced cytotoxic effects. Instead, EGF-PE40 led to a nearly complete inhibition of protein biosynthesis in the PCa cells and to a time-dependent cytotoxicity with IC_{50} values in the low nanomolar to picomolar range. EGF-PE24mut led to IC_{50} values in the single-digit nanomolar range and was thus significantly less toxic than EGF-PE40. As a cause we found a lower inhibition of protein biosynthesis by EGF-PE24mut compared to the PE40-based immunotoxin. Further investigations need to show if this is due to a reduced cytosolic uptake, since the translocation domain is completely deleted in PE24mut with exception of the furin cleavable site. Overall, the C4-2 and PC-3 cells proved to be less sensitive to the targeted toxins than the LNCaP cells. Not all cells of these lines were killed within a time period of 72 h and the cleavage of caspase-3 and PARP was not as pronounced as in LNCaP cells. Therefore, further investigations are needed to determine whether the targeted toxins did not enter the cytosol sufficiently due to increased lysosomal or proteasomal degradation or other obstacles during trafficking, or whether there is increased apoptosis resistance against the targeted toxins in these two cell lines.

The cytotoxicity of our targeted toxins are comparable with those of Niesen and colleagues, that consisted of the anti-EGFR scFv 2112 from Cetuximab or the anti-EGFR scFv 1711 from Panitumumab and ETA′, a truncated version of PE. Both showed a high cytotoxicity on the PCa cell line C4-2 with IC_{50} values of 55 pm for scFv2112-ETA′ and 192 pM for scFv1711-ETA′ after 72 h, respectively [29].

Despite a reduced cytotoxicity compared to our PE40-based immunotoxin, EGF-PE24mut should be more suitable for use in patients than EGF-PE40 due to its lack of immunogenicity. Moreover, it was still proven to be at least 600 to 3000-fold more cytotoxic than the EGFR inhibitor erlotinib, which mostly failed in clinical studies with patients suffering from PCa [24,26]. The increased cytotoxicity of our targeted toxins compared to inhibitors, like erlotinib, can be attributed to their enzymatic ADP-ribosyltransferase activity. Thus, only a few toxin molecules are sufficient to inhibit the protein biosynthesis of the target cells to such an extent that apoptosis is triggered. With competitive inhibitors, such as erlotinib, however, only a stoichiometric one to one binding can result in receptor tyrosine kinase blocking.

Since EGFR is also expressed on normal cells, it cannot be excluded that the treatment of PCa patients with our targeted toxins could lead to side effects due to on-target/off-tumor activities. It is therefore conceivable that in the future a combination therapy would be helpful with drugs that are directed against, for example PSMA, which is largely expressed on PCa cells and mostly organ-specific [43]. It appears to be reasonable to overcome the reduced efficiency of EGF-PE24mut because the minimized immunogenicity of this fusion protein is a substantial advantage for clinical applications. Testing of our targeted toxins in mouse models is required in the future with regard to reduced immunogenicity versus antitumor activity. Diminished cytosolic uptake due to the lack of the toxin's intrinsic domain required to support membrane transfer might be compensated by strategies described to temporarily weaken the membrane integrity comprising lysosomotropic amines, carboxylic ionophores and calcium channel antagonists [44]. The most promising techniques in this regard include the use of cell-penetrating peptides [45], light-induced techniques [46] and co-application of glycosylated triterpenoids [47].

In summary, we could show that PE-based targeted toxins with the EGF ligand as binding domain are promising candidates for the treatment of prostate cancer. By using this human ligand and the de-immunized PE24mut toxin domain, the potential risk of immunogenicity in PCa patients could be diminished in the future.

4. Materials and Methods

4.1. Cells and Chemicals

The EGFR-expressing human PCa cell lines LNCaP, DU145, ad PC-3 were obtained from the American Type Culture Collection (ATCC, Manassas, VA, USA). Cell line identity was verified by short tandem repeat (STR) analysis (CLS GmbH, Eppelheim, Germany). A Chinese hamster ovary (CHO) cell line with lack of human EGFR expression served as EGFR-negative control and was purchased from Gibco (Gibco, Invitrogen, Karlsruhe, Germany). LNCaP, DU145 and PC-3 cells were routinely propagated in complete RPMI 1640 medium, and CHO cells were propagated in complete F-12 medium (Gibco, Invitrogen, Karlsruhe, Germany), each with 10% fetal bovine serum (Biochrom, Berlin, Germany), penicillin (100 U/mL) and streptomycin (100 mg/L) as supplements, and incubated at 37 °C and 5% CO_2 to maintain exponential cell growth and proliferation. Erlotinib HCl (Selleck Chemicals Llc, Houston, TX, USA) was dissolved in DMSO as a 4 mg/mL stock solution, aliquoted and stored at −80 °C until use.

4.2. Cloning, Expression and Purification of EGF and the Anti-EGFR Immunotoxins

The human EGF ligand and the immunotoxins EGF-PE40, and EGF-PE24mut were cloned into the expression vector pHOG21 followed by chemical transformation of XL-1 blue supercompetent *E. coli* cells (Agilent Technologies, Santa Clara, CA, USA). Correct gene sequences were verified by gene sequencing (Microsynth Seqlab, Göttingen, Deutschland). The vector pHOG21 contains a 22 amino acid leader peptide (pel-B leader) at the N-terminus that directs the protein to the bacterial periplasm [48]. Periplasmatic expression and purification of EGF, EGF-PE40 and EGF-PE24mut via immobilized affinity chromatography (IMAC) were carried out as described earlier [49]. In brief, one successfully transformed bacteria clone each was inoculated over night at 37 °C in YT medium containing 0.1 M glucose and 100 mg/mL ampicillin. The following day, the culture was diluted 1:20 and grown in 600 mL medium until reaching an OD of 0.8, then pelleted by centrifugation and resuspended in 600 mL YT medium containing 50 mg/mL ampicillin, 0.4 M sucrose and 1 mM IPTG for overnight protein expression at RT. Bacteria cultures were centrifuged (6000 rpm, 4 °C, 10 min) and pellets were resuspended in 30 mL ice-cold Tris-HCl, 20% sucrose, 1 mM EDTA (pH 8.0) and incubated on ice for 1 h for the release of periplasmic proteins. For harvesting the periplasmatic extract, the suspension was centrifuged (10,000 rpm, 4 °C, 30 min) and supernatant was collected and dialyzed against 50 mM Tris-HCl, 1 M NaCl (pH 7.0). The periplasmatic extract (PE) was then purified with the help of HiTrap^{TM} Chelating High Performance columns with chelating sepharose (Sigma-Aldrich, St. Louis, MO, USA) charged with Ni^{2+} metal ions. Polyhistidine tagged EGF and immunotoxins were purified subsequently: The column was equilibrated with equilibration buffer [50 mM Tris-HCl, 1 M NaCl (pH 7.0)] and PE was loaded. Bound target proteins were eluted stepwise with varying imidazole concentrations of 40 mM (elution fraction E1), 80 mM (E2), and 250 mM (E3-5) and dialyzed against phosphate-buffered saline (PBS). Final protein yield of all preparations was determined by NanoDrop™ Lite Spectrophotometer (Thermo Fisher Scientific, Waltham, MA, USA).

4.3. Preparation of Cell Lysates

Target cells were lysed in RIPA buffer (50 nM Tris-HCl, 150 nM NaCl, 1 mM EDTA, 0.5% NaDeoxycholate, 0.05% SDS, 1% Igepal), supplemented with Protease Inhibitor Cocktail (Merck Millipore, Burlington, MA, USA) and Phosphatase Inhibitor Cocktail (Sigma-Aldrich, St. Louis, MO, USA), and incubated on ice for 30 min. After centrifugation (13,000 rpm, 4 °C, 30 min), the supernatant was collected and quantification of protein content was determined by Quick Start™ Bradford Protein Assay (Bio-Rad Laboratories, Inc., Hercules, CA, USA). The whole cell lysates were aliquoted and stored at −80 °C.

4.4. SDS-PAGE and Western Blot

SDS-PAGE and Western Blot were used to verify the expression and purification of EGF, EGF-PE40, and EGF-PE24mut according to previous descriptions [50]. Purified preparations were detected by HRP-conjugated c-myc mouse mAb (Roche Diagnostics, Mannheim, Germany, #11814150001). EGFR expression in the target cells was assessed by Western Blotting of whole cell lysate (50 µg per lane) with the help of EGFR rabbit pAb (Santa Cruz Biotechnology, Dallas, TX, USA, #sc-03) and HRP-labeled goat anti-rabbit pAb (Dako Denmark A/S, Glostrup, Denmark, #P0448).

Induction of apoptosis in the target cells was determined by Western Blot (50 µg per lane). Caspase-3 activation and poly-(ADP-ribose)polymerase (PARP) cleavage were detected by Cas-3 mouse mAb (ECM Biosciences, Versailles, KY, USA, #CM4911) and PARP rabbit pAb (Cell Signaling Technology Europe, Leiden, The Netherlands, #9542) as primary antibodies. HRP-labeled goat anti-rabbit pAb (Dako Denmark A/S, Glostrup, Denmark, #P0448) and HRP-labeled rabbit anti-mouse pAb (Dako Denmark A/S, Glostrup, Denmark, #P016) served as secondary antibodies.

β-Actin was used as a loading control and detected by HRP-conjugated β-Actin rabbit pAb (Cell Signaling Technology Europe, Leiden, The Netherlands, #5125). Visualization and analysis of protein bands was carried out by developing the membranes with an enhanced chemiluminescence (ECL) system (Clarity™ Western ECL Substrate, Bio-Rad Laboratories, Inc., Hercules, CA, USA), the ChemiDoc™ MP Imaging System and the software Image Lab™.

4.5. Flow Cytometry

Characterization of EGFR expression on the target cell surface was examined by flow cytometric analysis as described by us earlier [50]. PE-labeled EGFR mAb (BioLegend, San Diego, CA, USA, #352903) was used as detection antibody.

Binding of the EGF ligand, EGF-PE40, and EGF_PE24mut to EGFR on the target cells was confirmed by flow cytometry. Bound EGF and targeted toxins were detected via His-tag rabbit mAb (Cell Signaling Technology Europe, Leiden, The Netherlands, #12698) and goat anti-rabbit IgG-PE (Southern Biotech, Birmingham, AL, USA, #4010-09S). Mean fluorescence values of stained cells were determined with a FACS Calibur flow cytometer and the software CellQuest Pro (BD Biosciences, Heidelberg, Germany).

4.6. Inhibition of Protein Biosynthesis

For the verification of protein biosynthesis inhibition via Western Blot, cells were incubated with EGF-PE40 or EGF-PE24 at approx. IC_{20} concentrations of EGF-PE40 for 48 h (LNCaP) or 72 h (DU145, PC-3, CHO). Puromycin (5 µg/mL) (Tocris, Bio-Techne GmbH, Wiesbaden, Germany) was added to the cells 15 min before harvesting. RIPA lysate preparation was carried out as described above. Western Blot membranes were stained with puromycin mouse mAb (Merck Chemicals, Darmstadt, Germany, #MABE343) and HRP-labeled rabbit anti-mouse pAb (Dako Denmark A/S, Glostrup, Denmark, #P016).

4.7. WST-1 Cell Viability Assay

Cytotoxicity after immunotoxin treatment was quantified by the colorimetric WST-1-Assay according to the standard protocol (Roche Diagnostics). Based on the enzymatic cleavage of the water-soluble tetrazolium salt WST-1 (2–(4–Iodophenyl)–3–(4–nitrophenyl)–5-(2,4–disulfophenyl)–2H–tetrazolium, monosodium salt) to formazan, the number of metabolically active cells can be approximated proportionally.

4.8. Bright-Field Microscopy

Morphology of the target cells after treatment with EGF-PE40 and EGF-PE24mut was studied by bright-field microscopy using the confocal laser scanning microscope LSM 880 with Airyscan (Carl Zeiss Microscopy, Göttingen, Germany).

4.9. Statistical Analysis

Binding affinity of EGF was calculated by GraphPad Prism 7 software (GraphPad Software, San Diego, CA, USA). K_D values were defined as the drug concentrations leading to half-maximal specific binding. 50% inhibitory concentrations (IC_{50}) values of WST-1 data were calculated for the targeted toxins and erlotinib on each cell line using GraphPad Prism 7 software by non-linear regression ([inhibitor] vs. normalized response).

Supplementary Materials: The following are available online at http://www.mdpi.com/2072-6651/12/12/753/s1, Table S1. Binding of EGF and the targeted toxins EGF-PE40 and EGF-PE24mut to PC cells; Figure S1: Morphological changes of PCa cells upon treatment with EGF-based targeted toxins. Figure S2: Influence of the EGFR inhibitor erlotinib on the viability of PCa cells. Figure S3: Whole Western Blots including densitometry ratios.

Author Contributions: Conceptualization, A.P.M., P.W.; Resources, H.F., P.W.; Methodology, A.P.M., P.W.; Performance of experiments, A.F., A.P.M., I.W.; Validation, A.F., A.P.M., H.F., P.W.; Statistical analysis, A.F., A.P.M.; Writing—Original Draft Preparation, A.F., A.P.M., P.W.; Writing—Review & Editing, I.W., A.P.M., H.F., P.W.; Supervision, P.W.; Project Administration, P.W.; All authors have read and agreed to the published version of the manuscript

Funding: This research was supported by a grant of the German Research Foundation to P.W. (No. 2178/2-1). The article processing charge was funded by the Baden-Wuerttemberg Ministry of Science, Research and Art and the University of Freiburg in the funding programme "Open Access Publishing".

Acknowledgments: We thank I. Kuckuck and S. Schultze-Seemann for excellent technical assistance.

Conflicts of Interest: The authors declare no conflict of interest.

References

1. Bray, F.; Ferlay, J.; Soerjomataram, I.; Siegel, R.L.; Torre, L.A.; Jemal, A. Global cancer statistics 2018: Globocan estimates of incidence and mortality worldwide for 36 cancers in 185 countries. *CA Cancer J. Clin.* **2018**, *68*, 394–424. [CrossRef] [PubMed]
2. Litwin, M.S.; Tan, H.J. The diagnosis and treatment of prostate cancer: A review. *JAMA* **2017**, *317*, 2532–2542. [CrossRef] [PubMed]
3. Cha, H.R.; Lee, J.H.; Ponnazhagan, S. Revisiting immunotherapy: A focus on prostate cancer. *Cancer Res.* **2020**, *80*, 1615–1623. [CrossRef] [PubMed]
4. Fay, E.K.; Graff, J.N. Immunotherapy in prostate cancer. *Cancers* **2020**, *12*, 1752. [CrossRef] [PubMed]
5. Elsässer-Beile, U.; Bühler, P.; Wolf, P. Targeted therapies for prostate cancer against the prostate specific membrane antigen. *Curr. Drug Targets* **2009**, *10*, 118–125. [CrossRef] [PubMed]
6. Cimadamore, A.; Cheng, M.; Santoni, M.; Lopez-Beltran, A.; Battelli, N.; Massari, F.; Galosi, A.B.; Scarpelli, M.; Montironi, R. New prostate cancer targets for diagnosis, imaging, and therapy: Focus on prostate-specific membrane antigen. *Front. Oncol.* **2018**, *8*, 653. [CrossRef] [PubMed]
7. Yang, X.; Guo, Z.; Liu, Y.; Si, T.; Yu, H.; Li, B.; Tian, W. Prostate stem cell antigen and cancer risk, mechanisms and therapeutic implications. *Expert Rev. Anticancer Ther.* **2014**, *14*, 31–37. [CrossRef]
8. Antonarakis, E.S.; Carducci, M.A.; Eisenberger, M.A. Novel targeted therapeutics for metastatic castration-resistant prostate cancer. *Cancer Lett.* **2010**, *291*, 1–13. [CrossRef]

9. Lorenzo, G.D.; Bianco, R.; Tortora, G.; Ciardiello, F. Involvement of growth factor receptors of the epidermal growth factor receptor family in prostate cancer development and progression to androgen independence. *Clin. Prostate Cancer* **2003**, *2*, 50–57. [CrossRef]
10. Guérin, O.; Fischel, J.L.; Ferrero, J.M.; Bozec, A.; Milano, G. EGFR targeting in hormone-refractory prostate cancer: Current appraisal and prospects for treatment. *Pharmaceuticals* **2010**, *3*, 2238–2247. [CrossRef]
11. Burgess, A.W. Egfr family: Structure physiology signalling and therapeutic targets. *Growth Factors* **2008**, *26*, 263–274. [CrossRef]
12. Ogiso, H.; Ishitani, R.; Nureki, O.; Fukai, S.; Yamanaka, M.; Kim, J.H.; Saito, K.; Sakamoto, A.; Inoue, M.; Shirouzu, M.; et al. Crystal structure of the complex of human epidermal growth factor and receptor extracellular domains. *Cell* **2002**, *110*, 775–787. [CrossRef]
13. Ferguson, K.M. Structure-based view of epidermal growth factor receptor regulation. *Ann. Rev. Biophys.* **2008**, *37*, 353–373. [CrossRef] [PubMed]
14. Harris, R.C.; Chung, E.; Coffey, R.J. EGF receptor ligands. *Exp. Cell Res.* **2003**, *284*, 2–13. [CrossRef]
15. Wee, P.; Wang, Z. Epidermal growth factor receptor cell proliferation signaling pathways. *Cancers* **2017**, *9*, 52. [CrossRef]
16. Bonaccorsi, L.; Nosi, D.; Muratori, M.; Formigli, L.; Forti, G.; Baldi, E. Altered endocytosis of epidermal growth factor receptor in androgen receptor positive prostate cancer cell lines. *J. Mol. Endocrinol.* **2007**, *38*, 51–66. [CrossRef]
17. Day, K.C.; Lorenzatti Hiles, G.; Kozminsky, M.; Dawsey, S.J.; Paul, A.; Broses, L.J.; Shah, R.; Kunja, L.P.; Hall, C.; Palanisamy, N.; et al. Her2 and EGFR overexpression support metastatic progression of prostate cancer to bone. *Cancer Res.* **2017**, *77*, 74–85. [CrossRef]
18. DeHaan, A.M.; Wolters, N.M.; Keller, E.T.; Ignatoski, K.M. Egfr ligand switch in late stage prostate cancer contributes to changes in cell signaling and bone remodeling. *Prostate* **2009**, *69*, 528–537. [CrossRef]
19. Chang, Y.S.; Chen, W.Y.; Yin, J.J.; Sheppard-Tillman, H.; Huang, J.; Liu, Y.N. Egf receptor promotes prostate cancer bone metastasis by downregulating mir-1 and activating twist1. *Cancer Res.* **2015**, *75*, 3077–3086. [CrossRef]
20. De Muga, S.; Hernandez, S.; Agell, L.; Salido, M.; Juanpere, N.; Lorenzo, M.; Lorente, J.A.; Serrano, S.; Lloreta, J. Molecular alterations of EGFR and PTEN in prostate cancer: Association with high-grade and advanced-stage carcinomas. *Modern Pathol.* **2010**, *23*, 703–712. [CrossRef]
21. Di Lorenzo, G.; Tortora, G.; D'Armiento, F.P.; De Rosa, G.; Staibano, S.; Autorino, R.; D'Armiento, M.; De Laurentiis, M.; De Placido, S.; Catalano, G.; et al. Expression of epidermal growth factor receptor correlates with disease relapse and progression to androgen-independence in human prostate cancer. *Clin. Cancer Res.* **2002**, *8*, 3438–3444.
22. Schlomm, T.; Kirstein, P.; Iwers, L.; Daniel, B.; Steuber, T.; Walz, J.; Chun, F.H.; Haese, A.; Kollermann, J.; Graefen, M.; et al. Clinical significance of epidermal growth factor receptor protein overexpression and gene copy number gains in prostate cancer. *Clin. Cancer Res.* **2007**, *13*, 6579–6584. [CrossRef] [PubMed]
23. Hour, T.C.; Chung, S.D.; Kang, W.Y.; Lin, Y.C.; Chuang, S.J.; Huang, A.M.; Wu, W.J.; Huang, S.P.; Huang, C.Y.; Pu, Y.S. Egfr mediates docetaxel resistance in human castration-resistant prostate cancer through the akt-dependent expression of abcb1 (mdr1). *Arch. Toxicol.* **2015**, *89*, 591–605. [CrossRef] [PubMed]
24. Gravis, G.; Bladou, F.; Salem, N.; Gonçalves, A.; Esterni, B.; Walz, J.; Bagattini, S.; Marcy, M.; Brunelle, S.; Viens, P. Results from a monocentric phase ii trial of erlotinib in patients with metastatic prostate cancer. *Ann. Oncol.* **2008**, *19*, 1624–1628. [CrossRef] [PubMed]
25. Canil, C.M.; Moore, M.J.; Winquist, E.; Baetz, T.; Pollak, M.; Chi, K.N.; Berry, S.; Ernst, D.S.; Douglas, L.; Brundage, M.; et al. Randomized phase ii study of two doses of gefitinib in hormone-refractory prostate cancer: A trial of the national cancer institute of Canada-clinical trials group. *J. Clin. Oncol* **2005**, *23*, 455–460. [CrossRef] [PubMed]
26. Gross, M.; Higano, C.; Pantuck, A.; Castellanos, O.; Green, E.; Nguyen, K.; Agus, D.B. A phase ii trial of docetaxel and erlotinib as first-line therapy for elderly patients with androgen-independent prostate cancer. *BMC Cancer* **2007**, *7*, 142. [CrossRef] [PubMed]
27. Horti, J.; Widmark, A.; Stenzl, A.; Federico, M.H.; Abratt, R.P.; Sanders, N.; Pover, G.M.; Bodrogi, I. A randomized, double-blind, placebo-controlled phase ii study of vandetanib plus docetaxel/prednisolone in patients with hormone-refractory prostate cancer. *Cancer Biother. Radiopharm.* **2009**, *24*, 175–180. [CrossRef] [PubMed]

28. Cathomas, R.; Rothermundt, C.; Klingbiel, D.; Bubendorf, L.; Jaggi, R.; Betticher, D.C.; Brauchli, P.; Cotting, D.; Droege, C.; Winterhalder, R.; et al. Efficacy of cetuximab in metastatic castration-resistant prostate cancer might depend on egfr and pten expression: Results from a phase ii trial (sakk 08/07). *Clin. Cancer Res.* **2012**, *18*, 6049–6057. [CrossRef] [PubMed]
29. Niesen, J.; Stein, C.; Brehm, H.; Hehmann-Titt, G.; Fendel, R.; Melmer, G.; Fischer, R.; Barth, S. Novel egfr-specific immunotoxins based on panitumumab and cetuximab show in vitro and ex vivo activity against different tumor entities. *J. Cancer Res. Clinic. Oncol.* **2015**, *141*, 2079–2095. [CrossRef]
30. Wiley, H.S. Trafficking of the erbb receptors and its influence on signaling. *Exp. Cell Res.* **2003**, *284*, 78–88. [CrossRef]
31. Simon, N.; FitzGerald, D. Immunotoxin therapies for the treatment of epidermal growth factor receptor-dependent cancers. *Toxins* **2016**, *8*, 137. [CrossRef]
32. Yip, W.L.; Weyergang, A.; Berg, K.; Tønnesen, H.H.; Selbo, P.K. Targeted delivery and enhanced cytotoxicity of cetuximab-saporin by photochemical internalization in egfr-positive cancer cells. *Mol. Pharm.* **2007**, *4*, 241–251. [CrossRef] [PubMed]
33. Mazor, R.; Pastan, I. Immunogenicity of immunotoxins containing pseudomonas exotoxin a: Causes, consequences, and mitigation. *Front. Immunol.* **2020**, *11*, 1261. [CrossRef] [PubMed]
34. Liu, W.; Onda, M.; Lee, B.; Kreitman, R.J.; Hassan, R.; Xiang, L.; Pastan, I. Recombinant immunotoxin engineered for low immunogenicity and antigenicity by identifying and silencing human b-cell epitopes. *Proc. Natl. Acad. Sci. USA* **2012**, *109*, 11782–11787. [CrossRef] [PubMed]
35. Wolf, P.; Elsasser-Beile, U. Pseudomonas exotoxin a: From virulence factor to anti-cancer agent. *Int. J. Med. Microbiol.* **2009**, *299*, 161–176. [CrossRef] [PubMed]
36. Yarmolinsky, M.B.; Haba, G.L. Inhibition by puromycin of amino acid incorporation into protein. *Proc. Natl. Acad. Sci. USA* **1959**, *45*, 1721–1729. [CrossRef] [PubMed]
37. Nathans, D. Puromycin inhibition of protein synthesis: Incorporation of puromycin into peptide chains. *Proc. Natl. Acad. Sci USA* **1964**, *51*, 585–592. [CrossRef] [PubMed]
38. Russell, P.J.; Kingsley, E.A. Human prostate cancer cell lines. *Methods Mol. Med.* **2003**, *81*, 21–39.
39. Mazor, R.; Onda, M.; Pastan, I. Immunogenicity of therapeutic recombinant immunotoxins. *Immunol. Rev.* **2016**, *270*, 152–164. [CrossRef]
40. Azemar, M.; Schmidt, M.; Arlt, F.; Kennel, P.; Brandt, B.; Papadimitriou, A.; Groner, B.; Wels, W. Recombinant antibody toxins specific for erbb2 and egf receptor inhibit the in vitro growth of human head and neck cancer cells and cause rapid tumor regression in vivo. *Int. J. Cancer* **2000**, *86*, 269–275. [CrossRef]
41. Michalska, M.; Wolf, P. Pseudomonas exotoxin a: Optimized by evolution for effective killing. *Front. Microbiol.* **2015**, *6*, 963. [CrossRef] [PubMed]
42. Van Ness, B.G.; Howard, J.B.; Bodley, J.W. Adp-ribosylation of elongation factor 2 by diphtheria toxin. Nmr spectra and proposed structures of ribosyl-diphthamide and its hydrolysis products. *J. Biol. Chem.* **1980**, *255*, 10710–10716. [PubMed]
43. Ghosh, A.; Heston, W.D. Tumor target prostate specific membrane antigen (psma) and its regulation in prostate cancer. *J. Cell Biochem.* **2004**, *91*, 528–539. [CrossRef] [PubMed]
44. Fuchs, H.; Weng, A.; Gilabert-Oriol, R. Augmenting the efficacy of immunotoxins and other targeted protein toxins by endosomal escape enhancers. *Toxins* **2016**, *8*, 200. [CrossRef] [PubMed]
45. Kondow-McConaghy, H.M.; Muthukrishnan, N.; Erazo-Oliveras, A.; Najjar, K.; Juliano, R.L.; Pellois, J.P. Impact of the endosomal escape activity of cell-penetrating peptides on the endocytic pathway. *ACS Chem. Biol.* **2020**, *15*, 2355–2363. [CrossRef] [PubMed]
46. Jerjes, W.; Theodossiou, T.A.; Hirschberg, H.; Hogset, A.; Weyergang, A.; Selbo, P.K.; Hamdoon, Z.; Hopper, C.; Berg, K. Photochemical internalization for intracellular drug delivery. From basic mechanisms to clinical research. *J. Clin. Med.* **2020**, *9*, 528. [CrossRef]
47. Fuchs, H.; Niesler, N.; Trautner, A.; Sama, S.; Jerz, G.; Panjideh, H.; Weng, A. Glycosylated triterpenoids as endosomal escape enhancers in targeted tumor therapies. *Biomedicines* **2017**, *5*, 14. [CrossRef]
48. Kipriyanov, S.M.; Moldenhauer, G.; Little, M. High level production of soluble single chain antibodies in small-scale escherichia coli cultures. *J. Immunol. Methods* **1997**, *200*, 69–77. [CrossRef]

49. Wolf, P.; Alt, K.; Wetterauer, D.; Buhler, P.; Gierschner, D.; Katzenwadel, A.; Wetterauer, U.; Elsasser-Beile, U. Preclinical evaluation of a recombinant anti-prostate specific membrane antigen single-chain immunotoxin against prostate cancer. *J. Immunother.* **2010**, *33*, 262–271. [CrossRef]
50. Michalska, M.; Schultze-Seemann, S.; Bogatyreva, L.; Hauschke, D.; Wetterauer, U.; Wolf, P. In vitro and in vivo effects of a recombinant anti-psma immunotoxin in combination with docetaxel against prostate cancer. *Oncotarget* **2016**, *7*, 22531–22542. [CrossRef]

toxins

MDPI

Article

Cytotoxicity Effect of Quinoin, Type 1 Ribosome-Inactivating Protein from Quinoa Seeds, on Glioblastoma Cells

Rossella Rotondo [1,†], Sara Ragucci [2,†], Salvatore Castaldo [1], Maria Antonietta Oliva [1], Nicola Landi [2], Paolo V. Pedone [2], Antonietta Arcella [1,*,‡] and Antimo Di Maro [2,‡]

1 INM IRCCS Istituto Neurologico Mediterraneo NEUROMED, Via Atinense 18, 86077 Pozzilli, Italy; rossellaross1988@gmail.com (R.R.); castaldosal90@gmail.com (S.C.); mariaantonietta.oliva@neuromed.it (M.A.O.)

2 Department of Environmental, Biological and Pharmaceutical Sciences and Technologies (DiSTABiF), University of Campania "Luigi Vanvitelli", Via Vivaldi 43, 81100 Caserta, Italy; sara.ragucci@unicampania.it (S.R.); nicola.landi@unicampania.it (N.L.); paolovincenzo.pedone@unicampania.it (P.V.P.); antimo.dimaro@unicampania.it (A.D.M.)

* Correspondence: arcella@neuromed.it

† These authors contributed equally to this work.

‡ These authors share equal senior authorship.

Abstract: Ribosome-inactivating proteins (RIPs) are found in several edible plants and are well characterized. Many studies highlight their use in cancer therapy, alone or as immunoconjugates, linked to monoclonal antibodies directed against target cancer cells. In this context, we investigate the cytotoxicity of quinoin, a novel type 1 RIP from quinoa seeds, on human continuous and primary glioblastoma cell lines. The cytotoxic effect of quinoin was assayed on human continuous glioblastoma U87Mg cells. Moreover, considering that common conventional glioblastoma multiforme (GBM) cell lines are genetically different from the tumors from which they derive, the cytotoxicity of quinoin was subsequently tested towards primary cells NULU and ZAR (two cell lines established from patients' gliomas), also in combination with the chemotherapeutic agent temozolomide (TMZ), currently used in glioblastoma treatment. The present study demonstrated that quinoin (2.5 and 5.0 nM) strongly reduced glioblastoma cells' growth. The mechanisms responsible for the inhibitory action of quinoin are different in the tested primary cell lines, reproducing the heterogeneous response of glioblastoma cells. Interestingly, primary cells treated with quinoin in combination with TMZ were more sensitive to the treatment. Overall, our data highlight that quinoin could represent a novel tool for glioblastoma therapy and a possible adjuvant for the treatment of the disease in combination with TMZ, alone or as possible immunoconjugates/nanoconstructs.

Keywords: patient-derived glioblastoma cell lines; *Chenopodium quinoa* wild; ribosome-inactivating proteins; quinoin; temozolomide

Key Contribution: Data here reported are interesting since quinoin could represent a novel tool for cancer therapy and, in particular, a possible adjuvant for the treatment of glioblastoma with chemotherapeutic agents, alone or as a cytotoxic portion in immunoconjugates/nanoconstructs to tune its action.

Citation: Rotondo, R.; Ragucci, S.; Castaldo, S.; Oliva, M.A.; Landi, N.; Pedone, P.V.; Arcella, A.; Di Maro, A. Cytotoxicity Effect of Quinoin, Type 1 Ribosome-Inactivating Protein from Quinoa Seeds, on Glioblastoma Cells. *Toxins* **2021**, *13*, 684. https://doi.org/10.3390/toxins13100684

Received: 6 August 2021
Accepted: 22 September 2021
Published: 25 September 2021

1. Introduction

Ribosome-inactivating proteins (RIPs) are a group of toxins essentially retrieved in flowering plants [1]. These toxins are enzymes (N-glycosylase; EC: 3.2.2.22) able to remove a single adenine (A4324 in rat) located at a universally conserved stem and loop sequence on the large rRNA, known as the α-sarcin-ricin loop (SRL) [2]. The loss of this specific adenine causes conformational changes in the SRL structure, after which the EF-G (in prokaryotes) and eEF-2 (in eukaryotes) elongation factors are unable to interact with ribosomes during mRNA-tRNA translocation, blocking translocation during protein synthesis [3].

These enzymes are classically grouped into type 1 and type 2 RIPs based on the absence or presence of a quaternary structure. Indeed, type 1 RIPs are monomeric proteins (~30-kDa) with N-glycosylase activity while type 2 RIPs are dimeric proteins (~60-kDa) consisting of an enzymatic A-chain homologous to type 1 RIPs, linked through a disulphide bond to a B-chain with lectin properties [4]. Moreover, tetrameric protein types (A-B)2 reported in the *Sambucus* genus belonging to the family *Adoxaceae* [5] or proteolytic-activated enzymes retrieved in cereals, synthesized as inactive precursors [6], were found.

RIPs are isolated in different amounts from several plant tissues [7] and are identified in many orders belonging to angiosperms but not in gymnosperms [8,9]. Their physiological function in plants is still unknown, although it is associated with defense roles against herbivores, insects, fungi, and viruses [10]. This possible biological function is strengthened by the fact that several RIPs also have the ability to remove adenines from other substrates, such as RNAs and DNAs ('adenine polynucleotide glycosylases' activity), or have the capacity to cleave the phosphodiester bond (DNase activity [11]), which would amplify this function.

Research on RIPs had a great boost due to the potential biotechnological applications. In medicine, they are considered therapeutic agents against infected/tumor cells, due to the possible conjugation of type 1 or A-chain RIPs with antibodies (immunotoxins) or other carriers (peptides, specific proteins, or nanomaterials [12]) to obtain chimeric proteins able to direct these conjugates against specific targets [13,14]. In agriculture, RIPs could be employed as bio-pesticides to improve the resistance of cultivated plants towards insect, fungi, or viruses [10].

In acellular systems (*in vitro* translation), type 1 and type 2 RIPs display a similar toxicity, while in cellular systems, type 2 RIPs show higher toxicity (IC_{50} 0.0003–1.7 nM on Hela cells) with respect to type 1 (IC_{50} 170–3300 nM on Hela cells). In particular, the higher toxicity of type 2 RIPs is justified by the presence of the lectinic domain (B-chain), which possesses a strong affinity for sugar moieties on the cell surface, facilitating toxin entry into the cell [15]. Nevertheless, although less toxic, type 1 RIPs have a selective toxicity towards different cell lines, for which they could be potential drugs with clinical significance [15–17]. Moreover, RIPs cytotoxicity is correlated with the intracellular fate, considering the (i) expression of different types of ligands/receptors, (ii) cell surface and membrane composition (iii) routing of RIP-ligand complexes among different compartments, and (iv) availability of various pathways for transport of the A-chain into the cytosol [13].

In addition, type 1 RIPs, such as trichosanthin from *Trichosanthes kirilowii* [18,19] and saporin from *Saponaria officinalis* [20,21], display remarkable cytotoxicity against glioblastoma cell lines, which increases by linking them to specific conjugates [22]. This cytotoxicity is of interest, considering that glioblastoma is a highly aggressive brain tumor, in which malignant cells escape apoptosis by being resistant to radiotherapy and chemotherapy and unresponsive to drugs by rapidly inactivating or reducing intracellular drug concentrations or increasing the rate of DNA repair [23].

Recently, our group isolated and characterized a novel type 1 RIP from quinoa seeds, named quinoin, that displays cytotoxicity towards BJ-5ta (human fibroblasts) and HaCaT (human keratinocytes) in a dose- and time-dependent manner. Moreover, quinoin also exhibits a remarkable melting temperature (Tm ~ 68.2 °C), thermostability, and partial resistance proteolysis to cleavage [24]. These properties are of interest considering the possible use of quinoin as a natural drug alone or as an adjuvant to kill specific cells [25,26]. In this context, due to the great potential of quinoin as a toxin, we decided to test its cytotoxicity on glioblastoma cells.

Glioblastoma multiforme (GBM) is the most aggressive malignant primary brain tumor in humans, which remains incurable in most cases despite significant advances in therapy strategies [27]. GBM represents ~20% of all brain tumors and ~50% of all gliomas, being characterized by high proliferation, infiltration, and invasion, causing an objective difficulty to locally control GBM using radiotherapy or surgical excision [28].

Despite the progress in the field of neurosurgery and related treatment strategies, prognosis remains poor in most cases, with a median survival of ~14 months, due to therapeutic resistance and tumor recurrence after surgical removal, as well as tumor heterogeneity [28]. Currently, the standard GBM treatment includes maximum surgical excision, radiotherapy, and chemotherapy with temozolomide (TMZ), also known as temodal. The latter improves overall survival by ~2.5 months with respect to radiation alone, although it does not provide effective treatment of glioblastoma disease [28,29]. Therefore, we analyzed quinoin's effects on continuous U87Mg or primary NULU and ZAR glioblastoma cell lines, focusing our attention on the latter, whose heterogeneity reproduces the parental tumor from which it is derived [30]. Moreover, considering the pharmaco-resistant mechanisms of both tested primary cell lines to the alkylating agent TMZ [30], we verified the synergistic cytotoxic effect of quinoin in the presence of temodal on both NULU and ZAR cell lines.

On the other hand, some important limitations, such as blood-brain barrier impermeability, low rate of cell degeneration, inflammatory response, and activation of compensatory mechanisms, limit the use of RIPs alone [13]. Nevertheless, many RIPs-conjugates are used in cancer gene therapy considering their possible use as weapons against cancer cells. Indeed, several immunotoxins [17] or nanoconstructs [12] were obtained to make these toxins selective. Finally, RIPs-based toxins (chimeric molecules) have been designed as molecules in which the toxic domains are linked to selective tumor-targeting domains for cancer therapy.

A clear potential of this strategy is given by saporin-6, a type 1 RIP isolated from *Saponaria officinalis* seeds. This protein, similar to quinoin [31], is very used in several conjugates in neuroscience as a convenient tool to induce highly selective degeneration of a desired cell subpopulation. Indeed, saporin-based toxins, inducing selective cell death, are one of the approaches used to study (i) neurodegenerative diseases, (ii) the functions of certain cell subpopulations in the brain, and (iii) the development of alternative therapies [21].

In this scenario, considering the thermal stability and the resistance to proteolysis [24] of quinoin as well as its similarity to saporin-6, data reported in this work are a starting point for the possible use of quinoin as a novel therapeutic tool for current GBM treatment or as a novel tool in neuroscience.

2. Results

2.1. Quinoin Isolation

Quinoin was purified from the seeds of *C. quinoa* as previously reported [24]. The homogeneity of quinoin was achieved by both SDS-PAGE and RP-HPLC analysis (Figure S1) [32].

2.2. Inhibiting Effect of Quinoin on Cell Growth and Viability of Glioblastoma U87Mg and Patient-Derived Cell Lines NULU and ZAR

The inhibiting effect of quinoin occurs at a very low dose. This toxin is considered highly cytotoxic on both the U87Mg glioblastoma continuous cell line and primary cell lines NULU and ZAR as evidenced by the very low IC_{50} value (~5.0 nM). IC_{50} is the evaluation of the half-maximum inhibitory concentration of a substance and indicates the power of a drug to inhibit a specific biological or biochemical function by 50%. As reported in Figure 1, the IC_{50} values of GBM continuous and primary cells for quinoin did not exhibit a time dependence and the toxicity curves reached a plateau at high tested doses of the toxin. Similarly, what is reported in the breast cancer cell line MCF7 and glioblastoma cell line U87-Mg, type-II RIP Riproximin showed a recovery/resistance following longer exposure periods. Therefore, we can explain this interesting aspect with the assumption that a portion of the cell population developed a resistant mechanism to quinoin through the proposed mechanisms as previously reported [33].

	IC50-values (nM)		
	24h	48h	72h
Continuous cell line U87Mg	3.1 ± 2.2	4.6 ± 0.8	6.1 ± 0.8
Primary cell line NULU	6.6 ± 4.1	8.3 ± 1.6	2.3 ± 0.7
Primary cell line ZAR	3.4 ± 1.9	7.6 ± 2.7	3.3 ± 1.2

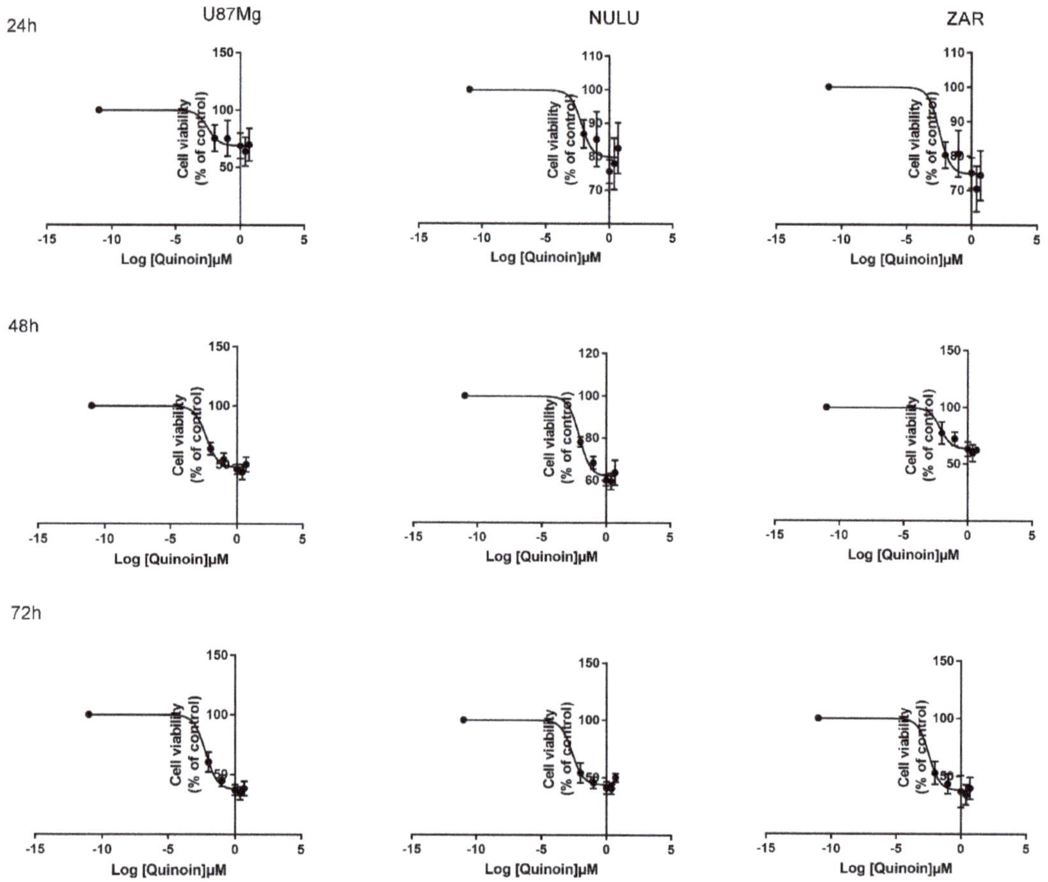

Figure 1. IC_{50} values estimation. IC_{50} values of U87Mg cells and two primary glioblastoma cell lines NULU and ZAR after 24, 48, and 72 h of incubation with quinoin using concentrations of 0.01, 0.1, 1.0, 2.5, and 5.0 µM. The control was assumed as part of the dose–response curve, considering it as a very low concentration (10^{-11} µM). Data were processed using GraphPad Prism and data are reported as Mean ± SD.

According to the IC_{50} value, we evaluated the effect of quinoin on human glioma cells growth rate, applying the drug at concentrations of 2.5 and 5.0 nM each day for a total of 3 days, starting one day after plating.

These treatments reduced the linear phase of growth in both the continuous cell line U87Mg and in primary glioblastoma cell lines (NULU and ZAR), with the cell number already being substantially reduced at 1 day after the beginning of the treatment and increased after two and three days (Figure 2A).

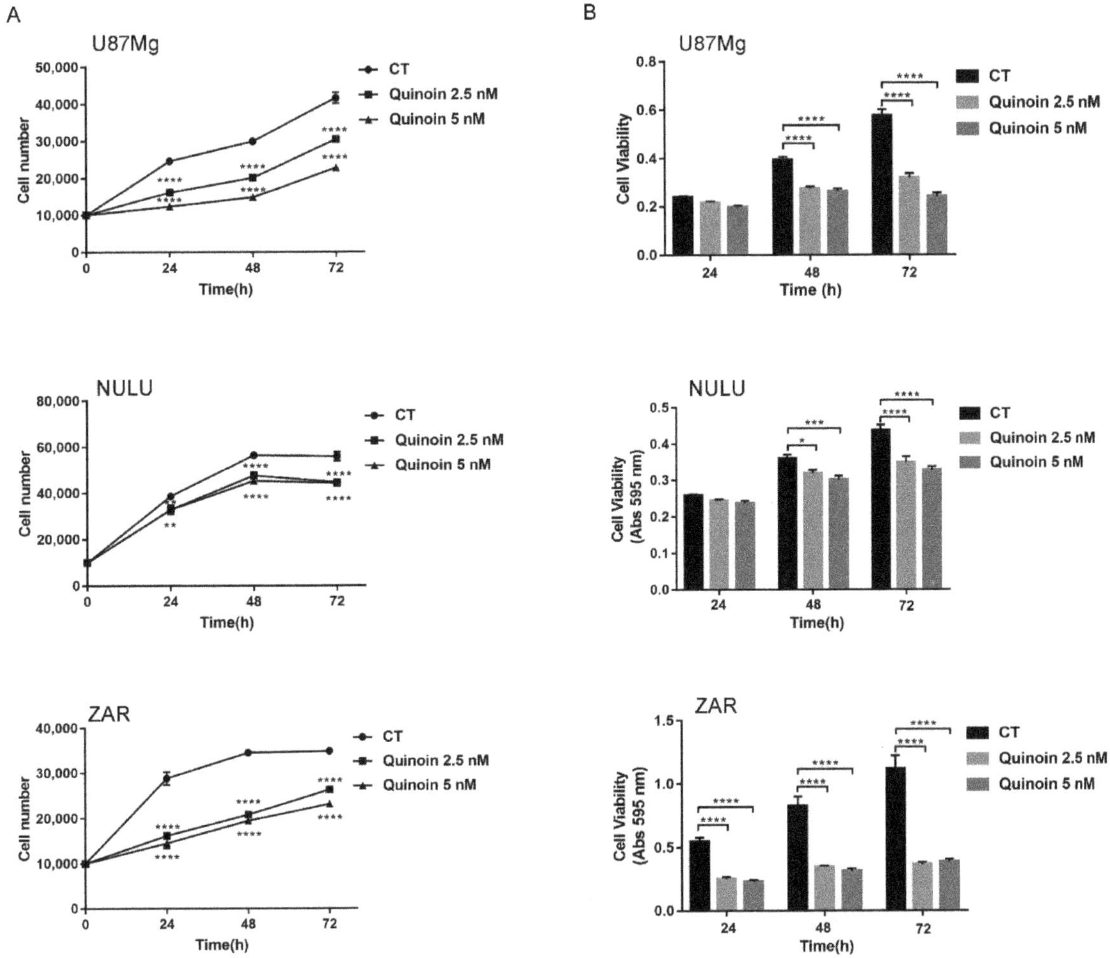

Figure 2. Growth curve and MTT assay of the U87Mg glioblastoma continuous cell line and primary cell lines. (**A**) On the left, the graphs of the growth curves of the continuous glioblastoma cell line U87Mg and of two primary cell lines obtained from the patient's biopsy (NULU and ZAR) are shown. Quinoin was administered at various doses of 2.5 and 5.0 nM daily, at various time intervals (1, 2, 3 days). (**B**) On the right, the graphs of the cell viability assessed by MTT assay. U87Mg and patient-derived glioblastoma cell lines NULU and ZAR treated daily with quinoin 2.5 and 5.0 nM, at various time intervals (1, 2, 3 days). Data shown are representative of three separate experiments and values are presented as Mean ± SEM. Statistical analysis was performed by one-way ANOVA. According to GraphPad Prism, * *p*-value 0.01 to 0.05 (significant), ** *p*-value 0.001 to 0.01 (very significant), *** *p*-value 0.0001 to 0.001 (extremely significant), **** *p*-value < 0.0001 (extremely significant).

The cytotoxicity of quinoin on glioblastoma cells, evaluated by MTT assay, revealed a significant reduction of the cell metabolic activity at concentrations of 2.5 and 5.0 nM. In particular, the primary cell line ZAR proved to be the most sensitive to quinoin treatment among the three glioblastoma cell lines, exhibiting a high response after 24 h of exposure (Figure 2B).

2.3. *Quinoin Treatment Results in Morphological Alteration in U87Mg Cells*

After 72 h of quinoin treatment at different concentrations (1.0, 2.5, and 5.0 μM), U87Mg cells revealed dramatic morphological changes by microscopic observation. The cells lost their polygonal shape and filaments, and cell shrinkage occurred to acquire a rounded phenotype typical of apoptotic cells (Figure 3).

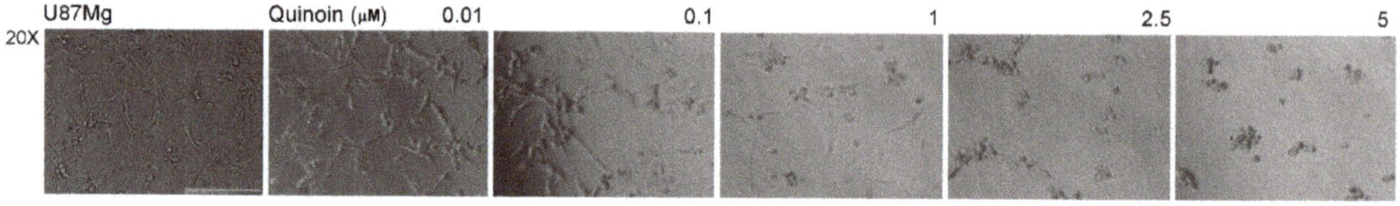

Figure 3. Morphological change of quinoin-treated U87Mg. The glioblastoma continuous cell line was exposed to 0.01, 0.1, 1.0, 2.5, and 5.0 μM quinoin for 72 h. Cells were imaged with an Evos FL microscope at 20× magnification.

The different response to quinoin treatment reflects the heterogeneous phenotype of primary glioblastoma cells.

Western blot analysis of patient-derived glioblastoma cells NULU treated with increasing concentrations of quinoin showed a dose-independent reduction of Cyclin D1 (Figures 4A and S2), while the ZAR cell line exhibited a significant reduction of Cyclin D1 at the maximal concentration used (250 nM) (Figure 4C).

Different responses of the primary cell lines to quinoin treatment were also revealed by investigating the activation of the apoptotic pathway. In this regard, the slight reduction of procaspase 3 in the NULU cell line was not detected in the ZAR cell line (Figure 4B,D).

The decrease of procaspase 3 was followed by a contemporary appearance of the activated form, which was visibly increased in the lysates of the cells treated with quinoin (Figure S3).

This heterogeneous response reflects the heterogeneous nature of primary glioblastoma cell lines, which faithfully reproduce the parental tumor from that they are derived [30]. Since the potential arrest of the cell cycle and activation of apoptosis are not the lead mechanisms underlying the quinoin-mediated cytotoxicity in the ZAR cell line, the induction of autophagy was also investigated. However, the common markers of the autophagic pathway, p62 and LC3B, did not show a significant change (Figure 4E,F), leading us to exclude the involvement of autophagy in primary glioblastoma cells treated with quinoin.

2.4. *Quinoin and Oxidative Stress*

In order to clarify the molecular mechanism of quinoin's action, the involvement of oxidative stress in quinoin-induced cytotoxicity was investigated. However, pretreatment with the ROS scavenger NAC (3.0 mM) indicated that the cytotoxic effects of quinoin are not mediated by oxidative stress (Figure 5).

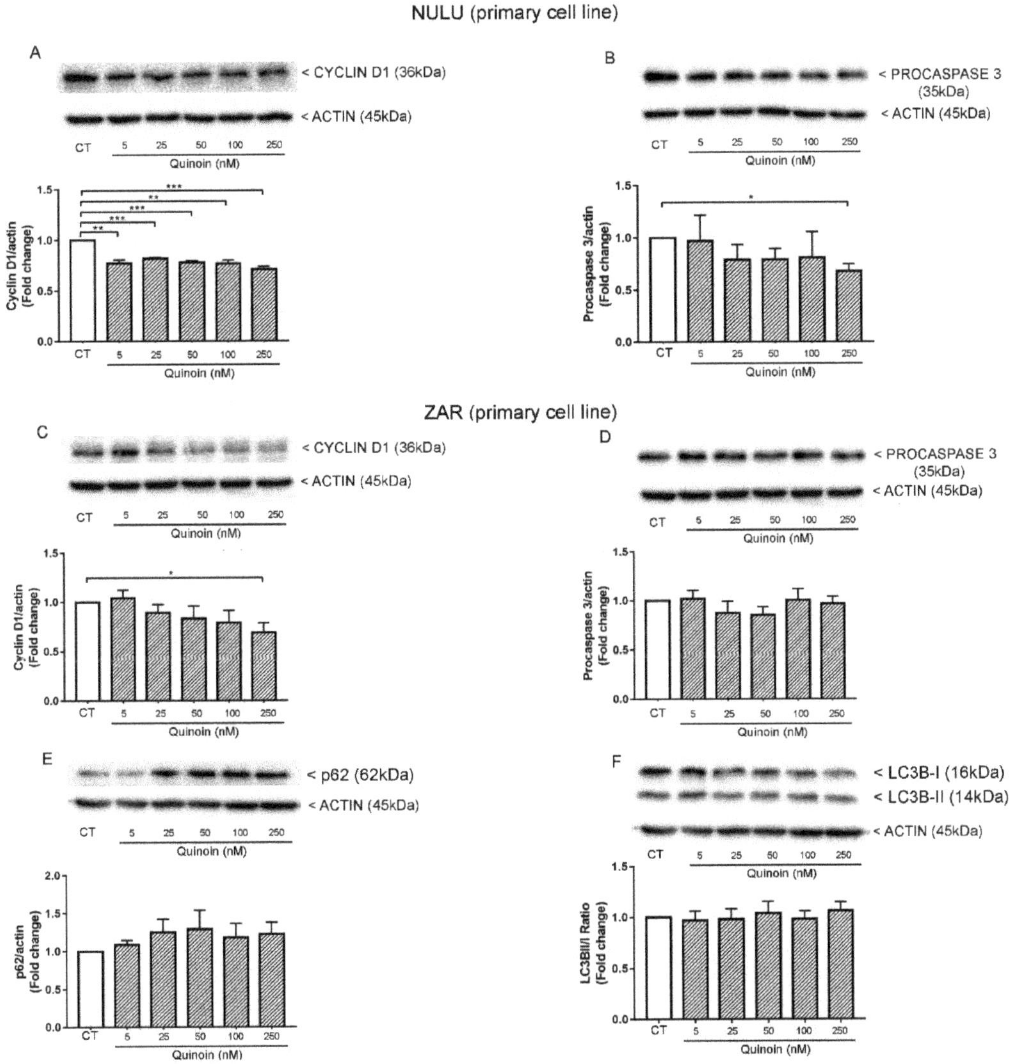

Figure 4. Western blot analysis of quinoin-treated primary cell lines for 24 h. (**A**) Quinoin induced a significant time-independent reduction of Cyclin D1 and (**B**) activation of apoptosis by a decrease of procaspase 3 when administered at a concentration of 250 nM in the NULU cell line. (**C**) Western blot analysis of the expression of Cyclin D1, (**D**) procaspase, and autophagic markers p62 (**E**) and LC3B (**F**) after treatment of the ZAR cell line with different concentrations of quinoin for 24 h. Densitometric analysis of protein levels represent the means ± SEM of three individual determinations. Data were normalized to the housekeeping gene actin and are expressed as a fold change over control-treated cells. * Unpaired *t*-test. According to GraphPad Prism, * *p*-value 0.01 to 0.05 (significant), ** *p*-value 0.001 to 0.01 (very significant), *** *p*-value 0.0001 to 0.001 (extremely significant).

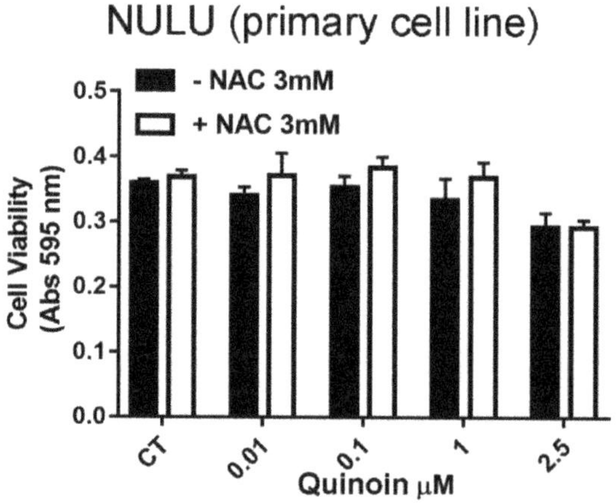

Figure 5. Quinoin and oxidative stress. Effect of primary cell line NULU's pre-treatment with the ROS scavenger NAC (3.0 mM) and evaluation of the cell viability under different concentrations of quinoin (0.01, 0.1, 1, and 2.5 μM) at 24 h from treatment. Data analyzed with the unpaired t-test revealed no significance.

2.5. *Quinoin as a Potential Adjuvant for Glioblastoma Treatment in Combination with Temozolomide*

Although the promoter of the O^6-methylguanine-methyltransferase (MGMT) gene was previously reported to be unmethylated in the primary cell lines NULU and ZAR [30], thus predicting potential TMZ resistance, the effective sensitivity to TMZ was verified by determining the IC_{50} value at 24 h. NULU, with an IC_{50} value of 8.4 ± 13.2 μM, was found to be more sensitive to TMZ with respect to ZAR (IC_{50} 141.8 ± 31.2 μM, Figure 6A).

A

	IC_{50} (μM) TMZ 24h
Primary GBM cell line NULU	8.4 ± 13.2
Primary GBM cell line ZAR	141.8 ± 31.2

B

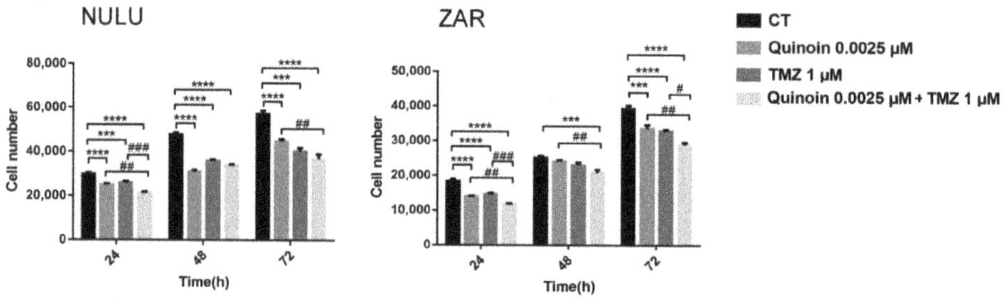

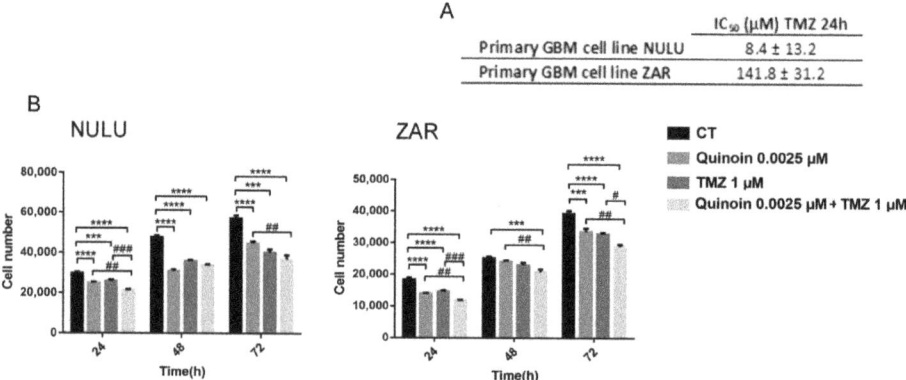

Figure 6. Combined treatment of quinoin and TMZ on primary glioblastoma cell lines. (**A**) IC_{50} values of TMZ of two primary glioblastoma cell lines, NULU and ZAR, after 24 h of incubation with TMZ. Data were processed using GraphPad Prism and data are reported as Mean ± SD. (**B**) Combined treatment in the presence of quinoin 2.5 nM and TMZ 1.0 μM for 24 h on NULU and ZAR primary cell lines. Data shown are representative of three separate experiments and values are presented as Mean ± SEM. Statistical analysis was performed by one-way ANOVA. According to GraphPad Prism, *** p-value 0.0001 to 0.001 (extremely significant), **** p-value < 0.0001 (extremely significant) significance vs. control cells; # p-value 0.01 to 0.05 (significant) significance of TMZ 1 μM vs. quinoin 2.5 nM plus TMZ 1.0 μM; ## p-value 0.001 to 0.01 (very significant) significance of quinoin 2.5 nM vs. quinoin 2.5 nM plus TMZ 1 μM; ### p-value 0.0001 to 0.001 (extremely significant) significance of TMZ 1 μM vs. quinoin 2.5 nM plus TMZ 1.0 μM.

The combination of quinoin (2.5 nM) with TMZ (1.0 μM) was found to be efficient in patient-derived GBM cell lines after 24 h of exposure (Figure 6B), indicating the potential of quinoin as a possible adjuvant in the treatment of glioblastoma.

3. Discussion

Glioblastoma is the most serious and common brain tumor affecting adults. It is malignant, infiltrating, expansive, and has a rapid growth pathology. These aspects, together with high angiogenesis, cellular heterogeneity, and the presence of a specific population of stem cells (brain tumor stem cells) that can proliferate and generate neoplastic glial cells [34], contribute to a poor prognosis: the median survival for this type of cancer is 14 months [28] with a 5-year survival rate of 2% [35].

There are numerous histopathological variants of GBM. In any case, features common to all types of GBM are cellular and nuclear pleomorphism, microvascular proliferation, and necrosis. In addition, GBM cells have an ability to activate numerous resistance mechanisms, complicating the search for effective therapy for this tumor. Among the pharmaco-resistant mechanisms to the alkylating agent (Temozolomide), the most common one found in GBM is O^6-methylguanine-methyltransferase (MGMT), a specific DNA repair protein, whose expression is variable due to the acquired methylation of the gene promoter during gliomagenesis. Despite the extensive surgical removal of what appears to be all microscopic diseases, either at the initial diagnosis or at the time of relapse, all patients will continue to show tumor growth and progression due to the rapid proliferation of infiltrative disease that persists after surgery. The current standard of care for the newly diagnosed disease includes maximum safe resection, followed by 6 weeks of concomitant daily radiotherapy and chemotherapy with temozolomide (TMZ) [28]. The addition of TMZ improves overall survival by ~2.5 months compared to radiation alone [29]. Notwithstanding attempts to improve outcomes for the newly diagnosed disease, effective treatment for glioblastoma remains unsolved. In this context, we assayed quinoin, type 1 RIP from quinoa seeds on a U87Mg continuous glioblastoma cell line and NULU and ZAR, two primary glioblastoma cell lines. Indeed, primary glioblastoma cell lines, developed from patients' biopsies, represent the genetic and histological features of patients [30]. The first experiment to evaluate quinoin IC_{50} revealed that this toxin shows high toxicity when glioblastoma cells were treated for 24, 48, and 72 h with concentrations ranging from 0.01 to 5.0 μM. The toxic effect of quinoin was evaluated on primary cell lines too, revealing the same toxicity profile. Moreover, the IC_{50} for all three glioblastoma cell lines did not decrease over time, indicating that quinoin toxicity is not time dependent. Therefore, we decided to use a single time point of 24 h for further experiments. The treatment with various toxin concentrations determined clear morphological change in U87Mg. Indeed, starting from quinoin 1.0 μM, the cells acquired a round form typical of apoptotic cells to reach a maximum effect at 5.0 μM (Figure 3). At this concentration, cells are completely rounded and without extensions. Moreover, growth curves at 1, 2, and 3 days after treatment with quinoin 2.5 or 5.0 nM displayed a statistically significant growth reduction, already at 1 day of treatment (Figure 2A), while MTT analysis in the same conditions reflected the trend of the growth curves (Figure 2B).

On the other hand, the common conventional GBM cell lines (e.g., U87Mg, U251, T98G, and A172) are genetically far from primary tumors due to the high number of passages in culture [36,37], losing the heterogeneity of GBM cells. Thus, we decided to investigate quinoin's effect on patient-derived cell lines, which resemble the parental tumor and are commonly used as a GBM model [30].

The analysis by Western blot showed that quinoin reduced the expression levels of Cyclin D1 in patient-derived glioblastoma cells NULU and ZAR, assuming that according to other mechanisms of RIPs action, quinoin induced a cell cycle arrest in G1/S phase [20]. However, considering the heterogeneity of GBM, quinoin induced cleavage of procaspase 3 and thus the action of the apoptotic pathway in the NULU primary cell line but not in the ZAR primary cell line. In the above tested conditions, quinoin induced cell death by reducing the expression levels of Cyclin D1 in NULU, but other possible mechanisms must also be investigated in other cell lines at different concentrations of this toxin. Several authors report another possible mode of action triggered by RIP toxins involving either reactive oxygen species (ROS) or the autophagy pathway. Indeed, some RIPs act by a a mechanism that involves reactive oxygen species (ROS) production in response to stress and increased intracellular calcium levels (e.g., abrin, trichosanthin) while, vice versa, other RIPs induce autophagy (e.g., gelonin, trichosanthin, and elderberry RIPs [17,38–40]). In this context, we evaluated the proteins involved in the autophagic process LC3BII/LC3BI and p62, which did not change when glioblastoma cells were treated with quinoin. Furthermore, quinoin cytotoxicity is not mediated by oxidative stress, since the pre-treatment with NAC 3.0 mM did not provide protection from quinoin's effects. These data reported here represent only the features of an innovative point of view to treat glioblastoma cell lines. The choice to investigate these genes (Cyclin D1, Caspase 3, p62, and LC3B) was suggested on the basis of literature, in which analogue pathways were investigated [20,40,41] for RIP proteins, such as saporin-6, tested on glioblastoma cell lines, GL15 and U87MG. Finally, we analyzed the effect of quinoin on glioblastoma cells' growth in the presence of canonical TMZ chemotherapy. The two drugs were combined according to the IC_{50} for TMZ and quinoin on both primary cell lines. Figure 6 highlights that in the presence of temodal, quinoin can determine a synergistic effect on both primary cell lines examined (NULU and ZAR), which exhibit a particular pharmaco-resistance due to the MGMT promoter unmethylation status [30]. To characterize the synergism between temodal and quinoin, we decided to test a lower concentration of quinoin (0.0025 µM) and Temodal (1.0 µM), thus making evaluation of the synergistic effects normally expected possible.

The synergistic interactions between the two drugs allow a reduction of the doses of the single drugs, obtaining in any case a complete therapeutic effect. The ability to predict this type of pharmacological function is therefore important because it helps to decrease toxicity and side effects. In this case, quinoin could also overcome drug resistance in glioblastoma cells, as drug resistance is responsible in most cases for the failure of drug therapy and early death of the patient [42]. This gives hope that quinoin could be used as an adjuvant drug at very low concentrations, given the high toxicity of the protein, although therapy with RIPs, capable of damaging protein synthesis in a non-discriminatory manner, cannot be considered without engineering the RIPs to target it only versus cancer cells.

Overall, quinoin exhibits cytotoxic action on both the U87Mg glioblastoma continuous cell line and primary cell lines NULU and ZAR and a synergic effect when used with Temozolomide. On the other hand, like other RIPs, quinoin is likely non-selective, probably presenting important limitations, such as blood-brain barrier impermeability, low rate of cell degeneration, inflammatory response, and activation of compensatory mechanisms that limit the use of RIPs alone [13]. These limitations can be overcome by toxin-conjugates considering their possible use as weapons against different cancer cells. Indeed, several immunotoxins [17] or nanoconstructs [12] were obtained to make RIPs selective.

In this framework, quinoin, similar to saporin-6 [21,24,31], is an attractive archetype of this toxin family and could represent a novel tool in biomedicine. Data reported in this work are the starting point for its possible use in neuroscience and in tumor therapy. Finally, since we cannot completely exclude that quinoin is able to pass through the blood-brain barrier, further experiments will be carried out, considering that the blood-brain barrier is disrupted in patients affected by glioblastoma [43,44].

4. Materials and Methods

4.1. Materials

Chemicals and chromatography for quinoin purification and the set-up conditions for RP-HPLC and SDS-PAGE analysis were obtained as previously reported [24].

4.2. Quinoin Purification

Native quinoin was purified from the seeds of white quinoa (*Chenopodium quinoa* Wild) as previously described [24] using a general protocol for the preparation of type 1 ribosome-inactivating proteins [32]. Determination of the protein concentration was achieved using the BCA colorimetric assay [ThermoFisher Scientific, Rodano (MI), Italy].

4.3. Cell Culture

The U87Mg human GBM cell lines were obtained from the Sigma Aldrich Collection (LGC Promochem, Teddington, UK). Cells were grown in Dulbecco's modified Eagle medium (DMEM) with the addition of 10% fetal bovine serum (FBS), 2 mmol/L-glutamine, 100 IU/mL penicillin, and 100 μg/mL streptomycin at 37 °C, 5% CO_2, and 95% humidity.

Human glioblastoma primary cell cultures were obtained from bioptic samples surgically removed from patients, who gave informed consent to participate in the study. The use of primary cell lines as a model for GBM heterogeneity was approved by Ethics Committee on 27 February 2020 and registered on ClinicalTrials.gov with the identification number NCT04180046. Samples were labelled using a three-letter code. After mechanical dissociation, single cells were resuspended in DMEM medium and centrifuged at 1200 RPM for 5 min. The pellet was resuspended in DMEM medium supplemented with 10% FBS and cells were plated on Petri plates (Falcon Primaria, Lincoln Park, NJ, USA). The medium was then changed every 3 days. After 14–15 days, cells were trypsinised, and re-plated into 24-well plates at a density of 25×10^3 cells/well. The established patient-derived GBM cell lines have been characterized and the genetic profile was previously reported [30].

4.4. IC_{50} Estimation of Quinoin and Temozolomide in U87Mg and Patient-Derived GBM Cell Lines

U87Mg cells and primary cell lines NULU and ZAR were plated in 96 wells with a density of 5×10^3 cells/well. The IC_{50} values of quinoin were determined at 24, 48, and 72 h using the MTT assay at concentrations of 0.01, 0.1, 1.0, 2.5, and 5.0 μM. In the same way, the IC_{50} value after 24 h of conventional chemotherapy with TMZ was determined in patient-derived glioblastoma cells NULU and ZAR, using TMZ concentrations of 10, 50, 100, 150, and 200 μM. Data were processed using GraphPad Prism (GraphPad Software Inc., San Diego, CA, USA) (https://www.graphpad.com/guides/prism/latest/curve-fitting/reg_50_of_what__relative_vs_absolu.htm; accessed on 21 September 2021) assuming the control as part of the dose–response curve, considering it as a very low concentration (10^{-11} μM).

4.5. Proliferation Assay

In order to evaluate the response to quinoin, U87Mg and patient-derived GBM cell lines were plated in 48 wells at a density of 1×10^4 cells/well in DMEM with 10% FBS, incubating them at a temperature of 37 °C with 5% of CO_2. On the basis of the IC_{50} values, cells were then treated daily with quinoin at established concentrations of 2.5 and 5.0 nM for 24, 48, and 72 h. The cell count was then performed using a Burker chamber.

4.6. Cell Viability Test

U87Mg and patient-derived GBM cell lines were plated in 96 wells at a density of 5×10^3 cells/well and treated daily for 24, 48, and 72 h at quinoin concentrations of 2.5 and 5.0 nM. The MTT assay (3-(4,5-dimethylthiazol-2-yl)-2,5-diphenyltetrazolium) (Sigma Chemical Co., St. Louis, MO, USA) was then performed. Specifically, 5 mg/mL of MTT were added to 100 μL of cells cultured in DMEM. The formazan crystals were dissolved with 0.4% isopropanol/HCl and the absorbance was measured at 595 nm with a plate reading spectrophotometer. To evaluate whether quinoin caused oxidative stress, primary GBM NULU cells were plated at a density of 5×10^3 cells/well and starved for 48 h in DMEM with 0.5% FBS. Cells were then pre-treated with the antioxidant N-acetylcysteine

(NAC) 3.0 mM for 4 h at 37 °C in DMEM with 10% FBS. The medium was replaced, and the cells were treated with quinoin at concentrations of 0.01, 0.1, 1.0, and 2.5 μM.

4.7. Microscopic Observation of Live Cells

U87Mg cells were plated in 96 wells in DMEM and 10% FBS and treated with 0.01, 0.1, 1.0, 2.5, and 5.0 μM of quinoin for 72 h. After treatment, the cells were observed with a phase contrast microscope (Evos, Life technologies, Monza, Italy) and morphological changes were evaluated.

4.8. Combined Treatment with TMZ and Quinoin

Primary GBM cell lines NULU and ZAR were plated in 48 wells at a density of 1×10^4 cells/well and treated with TMZ 1.0 μM either alone or in combination with quinoin 2.5 nM for 24, 48, and 72 h. After each treatment, the cells were counted through a Burker chamber.

4.9. Western Blot Analysis of U87Mg Cells Treated with Quinoin

In order to determine the protein expression in glioblastoma quinoin-treated cells, an extraction was performed with Triton X-100 lysis buffer (10 mM Tris•Cl, 1.0 mM EDTA, 150 mM NaCl, 1% Triton X-100, NaF 1.0 mM, 1.0 mM $Na_4P_2O_7$, 1.0 mM Na_3VO_4 and 1× protease inhibitors). Following the lysis, the extracted proteins (15 μg) were separated by 12.5% SDS-PAGE and transferred to PVDF membranes by electroblotting. The membranes were first saturated and incubated for 1 h at room temperature with 5% non-fat dry milk or BSA (bovine serum albumin) diluted in Tris 1× buffered saline containing Tween-20 (TBST), and subsequently incubated with specific primary antibodies overnight at 4 °C. Each membrane was also incubated with mouse monoclonal anti-β-actin (1: 10,000, Santa Cruz Biotechnology, Dallas, TX, USA) for protein normalization. The membranes were then exposed to secondary antibodies conjugated with the HRP enzyme (Calbiochem, Merk Life Science Srl., Milan, Italy). The protein bands were visualized by the chemiluminescence process using ECL Western blotting (GE healthcare Life Sciences, Milan, Italy), while the digital signals were quantified by densitometric analysis using the Image Lab software (Bio-Rad Laboratories, Rome, Italy).

To monitor the expression of the cell cycle protein Cyclin D1, the apoptotic protein procaspase 3, and the autophagic proteins p62 and LC3B, cells were plated at a density of 5×10^5 cells in 60 mm plates in DMEM (without FBS) and incubated for 48 h. After adding 10% FBS, cells were treated with different concentrations of quinoin (5.0, 25, 50,100, and 250 nM) for 24 h. The membranes were incubated with the antibodies anti-p62 and anti-LC3B (1:1000, Cell Signaling Technology, Euroclone, Pero, Italy), anti-Caspase 3 (1:1000, Cell Signaling Technology), and anti-Cyclin D1 (1:1000, Cell Signaling Technology).

4.10. Statistical Analysis

Data obtained from the experiments performed in triplicate are expressed as mean ± SEM and were analyzed by Student's-*t* test or one-way ANOVA. The differences were considered significant for $p < 0.05$. Analyses were carried out using the GraphPad Prism (GraphPad Software Inc.).

5. Conclusions

Until now, the effective treatment of glioblastoma disease represents one of the most important challenges for researchers. Moreover, poor prognosis, mainly due to therapeutic resistance and tumor recurrence after surgical removal, as well as tumor heterogeneity, have complicated the search for an effective glioblastoma therapy. On the other hand, the chemotherapeutic agent TMZ, used in current glioblastoma treatment, improves overall survival, although it does not provide an effective treatment for the disease. In this context, we investigated the cytotoxicity of quinoin, a novel type 1 RIP from quinoa seeds, on human continuous and primary glioblastoma cell lines while also evaluating the effect of this toxin towards primary cells, also in combination with TMZ. Interestingly, these findings suggest that RIPs could represent a novel effective strategy for glioblastoma therapy and a possible adjuvant for the treatment of the disease in combination with TMZ.

Overall, this study reveals that quinoin is a novel attractive tool in glioblastoma research that can counteract the growth of these cancer cells. In addition, the synergic effect of this toxin with canonical chemotherapy opens the way to possible uses of this toxin in strategies providing for its use in immunoconjugates or nanoconstructs to minimize the adverse effects in vivo when this toxin is used alone.

Supplementary Materials: The following are available online at https://www.mdpi.com/article/10.3390/toxins13100684/s1, Figure S1: (A) SDS-PAGE analysis of the purified quinoin with or without β-mercaptoethanol (lanes 1–2 and 3–4; 3.0 and 6.0 μg, respectively; M, protein markers). SDS-PAGE was carried out in 12% polyacrylamide separating gel. (B) Elution profile of purified quinoin by RP-HPLC. Quinoin (100 μg) was separated on a C4 column (Phenomenex, 0.46 × 25 cm), using a Waters Breeze HPLC system. The elution system contained 0.1% trifluoroacetic acid (TFA) in H_2O (solvent A) and 0.1% TFA in acetonitrile (solvent B). A gradient elution system was applied from 5% to 65% of solvent B in 60 min at a flow rate of 1.0 mL/min. Figure S2: Western Blot analysis of Cyclin D1 in primary glioblastoma cell lines NULU (A) and ZAR (B) treated with Quinoin 2.5 nM for 24, 48, and 72 h. Figure S3: Western blot analysis of Caspase 3 in primary glioblastoma cells NULU treated with Quinoin 5, 25, 50, 100, and 250 nM for 24 h. The blot revealed the presence of activated form of caspase 3.

Author Contributions: R.R., S.R., S.C., M.A.O. and N.L.: conducted the experiments. P.V.P., A.A. and A.D.M.: conceptualization, data analysis, writing and funding acquisition. All authors have read and agreed to the published version of the manuscript.

Funding: This research was funded by Italian Ministry of Health with Ricerca Corrente and the "Progetti per la ricerca oncologica della Regione Campania" (Grant: I-Cure). The APC was funded by IRCCS Neuromed and University of Campania "Luigi Vanvitelli".

Institutional Review Board Statement: The study was conducted according to the guidelines of the Declaration of Helsinki, and approved by the Ethics Committee of IRCCS Istituto Neurologico Mediterraneo NEUROMED (date of approval 27 February 2020).

Informed Consent Statement: Informed consent was obtained from all subjects involved in the study. The patients' biopsies were obtained from Neurosurgery department at IRCCS Neuromed. The use of primary cell lines as model for GBM heterogeneity was registered on ClinicalTrials.gov with identification number NCT04180046.

Data Availability Statement: The data presented in this study are available on request from the corresponding author.

Acknowledgments: This study was made possible by care and abnegation of all participants, despite the absence of dedicated funds and chronic difficulties afflicting the Italian scientific community.

Conflicts of Interest: The authors declare no conflict of interest.

References

1. Stirpe, F. Ribosome-inactivating proteins: From toxins to useful proteins. *Toxicon* **2013**, *67*, 12–16. [CrossRef]
2. Endo, Y.; Tsurugi, K. RNA N-glycosidase activity of ricin A-chain. Mechanism of action of the toxic lectin ricin on eukaryotic ribosomes. *J. Biol. Chem.* **1987**, *262*, 8128–8130. [CrossRef]
3. Shi, X.; Khade, P.K.; Sanbonmatsu, K.Y.; Joseph, S. Functional role of the sarcin-ricin loop of the 23S rRNA in the elongation cycle of protein synthesis. *J. Mol. Biol.* **2012**, *419*, 125–138. [CrossRef] [PubMed]
4. Barbieri, L.; Battelli, M.G.; Stirpe, F. Ribosome-inactivating proteins from plants. *Biochim. Biophys. Acta* **1993**, *1154*, 237–282. [CrossRef]
5. Tejero, J.; Jiménez, P.; Quinto, E.J.; Cordoba-Diaz, D.; Garrosa, M.; Cordoba-Diaz, M.; Gayoso, M.J.; Girbés, T. Elderberries: A source of ribosome-inactivating proteins with lectin activity. *Molecules* **2015**, *20*, 2364–2387. [CrossRef] [PubMed]
6. De Zaeytijd, J.; Van Damme, E.J. Extensive Evolution of Cereal Ribosome-Inactivating Proteins Translates into Unique Structural Features, Activation Mechanisms, and Physiological Roles. *Toxins* **2017**, *9*, 123. [CrossRef]
7. Park, S.W.; Lawrence, C.B.; Linden, J.C.; Vivanco, J.M. Isolation and characterization of a novel ribosome-inactivating protein from root cultures of pokeweed and its mechanism of secretion from roots. *Plant Physiol.* **2002**, *130*, 164–178. [CrossRef] [PubMed]

8. Di Maro, A.; Citores, L.; Russo, R.; Iglesias, R.; Ferreras, J.M. Sequence comparison and phylogenetic analysis by the Maximum Likelihood method of ribosome-inactivating proteins from angiosperms. *Plant Mol. Biol.* **2014**, *85*, 575–588. [CrossRef] [PubMed]
9. Lapadula, W.J.; Ayub, M.J. Ribosome Inactivating Proteins from an evolutionary perspective. *Toxicon* **2017**, *136*, 6–14. [CrossRef]
10. Zhu, F.; Zhou, Y.K.; Ji, Z.L.; Chen, X.R. The Plant Ribosome-Inactivating Proteins Play Important Roles in Defense against Pathogens and Insect Pest Attacks. *Front. Plant Sci.* **2018**, *9*, 146. [CrossRef]
11. Aceto, S.; Di Maro, A.; Conforto, B.; Siniscalco, G.G.; Parente, A.; Delli Bovi, P.; Gaudio, L. Nicking activity on pBR322 DNA of ribosome inactivating proteins from Phytolacca dioica L. leaves. *Biol. Chem.* **2005**, *386*, 307–317. [CrossRef]
12. Pizzo, E.; Di Maro, A. A new age for biomedical applications of Ribosome Inactivating Proteins (RIPs): From bioconjugate to nanoconstructs. *J. Biomed. Sci.* **2016**, *23*, 54. [CrossRef] [PubMed]
13. de Virgilio, M.; Lombardi, A.; Caliandro, R.; Fabbrini, M.S. Ribosome-inactivating proteins: From plant defense to tumor attack. *Toxins* **2010**, *2*, 2699–2737. [CrossRef]
14. Rust, A.; Partridge, L.J.; Davletov, B.; Hautbergue, G.M. The Use of Plant-Derived Ribosome Inactivating Proteins in Immunotoxin Development: Past, Present and Future Generations. *Toxins* **2017**, *9*, 334. [CrossRef] [PubMed]
15. Stirpe, F.; Gilabert-Oriol, R. Ribosome-Inactivating Proteins: An Overview. In *Plant Toxins*; Carlini, C.R., Ligabue-Braun, R., Gopalakrishnakone, P., Eds.; Springer: Dordrecht, The Netherlands, 2017; pp. 153–182.
16. Akkouh, O.; Ng, T.B.; Cheung, R.C.; Wong, J.H.; Pan, W.; Ng, C.C.; Sha, O.; Shaw, P.C.; Chan, W.Y. Biological activities of ribosome-inactivating proteins and their possible applications as antimicrobial, anticancer, and anti-pest agents and in neuroscience research. *Appl. Microbiol. Biotechnol.* **2015**, *99*, 9847–9863. [CrossRef] [PubMed]
17. Lu, J.Q.; Zhu, Z.N.; Zheng, Y.T.; Shaw, P.C. Engineering of Ribosome-inactivating Proteins for Improving Pharmacological Properties. *Toxins* **2020**, *12*, 167. [CrossRef]
18. Miao, J.; Jiang, Y.; Wang, D.; Zhou, J.; Fan, C.; Jiao, F.; Liu, B.; Zhang, J.; Wang, Y.; Zhang, Q. Trichosanthin suppresses the proliferation of glioma cells by inhibiting LGR5 expression and the Wnt/β-catenin signaling pathway. *Oncol. Rep.* **2015**, *34*, 2845–2852. [CrossRef]
19. Sha, O.; Yew, D.T.; Cho, E.Y.; Ng, T.B.; Yuan, L.; Kwong, W.H. Mechanism of the specific neuronal toxicity of a type I ribosome-inactivating protein, trichosanthin. *Neurotox. Res.* **2010**, *18*, 161–172. [CrossRef]
20. Cimini, A.; Mei, S.; Benedetti, E.; Laurenti, G.; Koutris, I.; Cinque, B.; Cifone, M.G.; Galzio, R.; Pitari, G.; Di Leandro, L.; et al. Distinct cellular responses induced by saporin and a transferrin-saporin conjugate in two different human glioblastoma cell lines. *J. Cell Physiol.* **2012**, *227*, 939–951. [CrossRef]
21. Bolshakov, A.P.; Stepanichev, M.Y.; Dobryakova, Y.V.; Spivak, Y.S.; Markevich, V.A. Saporin from Saponaria officinalis as a Tool for Experimental Research, Modeling, and Therapy in Neuroscience. *Toxins* **2020**, *12*, 546. [CrossRef]
22. Di Maro, A.; Pizzo, E.; Girbes, T. Biotechnological Potential of Ribosome-Inactivating Proteins (RIPs). In *Plant Toxins*; Carlini, C.R., Ligabue-Braun, R., Gopalakrishnakone, P., Eds.; Springer: Dordrecht, Netherlands, 2017; pp. 363–381.
23. Lah Turnšek, T.; Jiao, X.; Novak, M.; Jammula, S.; Cicero, G.; Ashton, A.W.; Joyce, D.; Pestell, R.G. An Update on Glioblastoma Biology, Genetics, and Current Therapies: Novel Inhibitors of the G Protein-Coupled Receptor CCR5. *Int. J. Mol. Sci.* **2021**, *22*, 4464. [CrossRef]
24. Landi, N.; Ruocco, M.R.; Ragucci, S.; Aliotta, F.; Nasso, R.; Pedone, P.V.; Di Maro, A. Quinoa as source of type 1 ribosome inactivating proteins: A novel knowledge for a revision of its consumption. *Food Chem.* **2021**, *342*, 128337. [CrossRef]
25. Santanché, S.; Bellelli, A.; Brunori, M. The unusual stability of saporin, a candidate for the synthesis of immunotoxins. *Biochem. Biophys. Res. Commun.* **1997**, *234*, 129–132. [CrossRef]
26. Tamburino, R.; Pizzo, E.; Sarcinelli, C.; Poerio, E.; Tedeschi, F.; Ficca, A.G.; Parente, A.; Di Maro, A. Enhanced cytotoxic activity of a bifunctional chimeric protein containing a type 1 ribosome-inactivating protein and a serine protease inhibitor. *Biochimie* **2012**, *94*, 1990–1996. [CrossRef] [PubMed]
27. Hanif, F.; Muzaffar, K.; Perveen, K.; Malhi, S.M.; Simjee Sh, U. Glioblastoma Multiforme: A Review of its Epidemiology and Pathogenesis through Clinical Presentation and Treatment. *Asian Pac. J. Cancer Prev. APJCP* **2017**, *18*, 3–9. [PubMed]
28. Stupp, R.; Mason, W.P.; van den Bent, M.J.; Weller, M.; Fisher, B.; Taphoorn, M.J.; Belanger, K.; Brandes, A.A.; Marosi, C.; Bogdahn, U.; et al. Radiotherapy plus concomitant and adjuvant temozolomide for glioblastoma. *N. Engl. J. Med.* **2005**, *352*, 987–996. [CrossRef] [PubMed]
29. Omar, A.I.; Mason, W.P. Temozolomide: The evidence for its therapeutic efficacy in malignant astrocytomas. *Core Evid.* **2010**, *4*, 93–111.
30. Oliva, M.A.; Staffieri, S.; Castaldo, S.; Giangaspero, F.; Esposito, V.; Arcella, A. Characterization of primary glioma cell lines derived from the patients according to 2016 CNS tumour WHO classification and comparison with their parental tumours. *J. Neurooncol.* **2021**, *151*, 123–133. [CrossRef]
31. Ragucci, S.; Bulgari, D.; Landi, N.; Russo, R.; Clemente, A.; Valletta, M.; Chambery, A.; Gobbi, E.; Faoro, F.; Di Maro, A. The Structural Characterization and Antipathogenic Activities of Quinoin, a Type 1 Ribosome-Inactivating Protein from Quinoa Seeds. *Int. J. Mol. Sci.* **2021**, *22*, 8964. [CrossRef]
32. Di Maro, A.; Valbonesi, P.; Bolognesi, A.; Stirpe, F.; De Luca, P.; Siniscalco Gigliano, G.; Gaudio, L.; Delli Bovi, P.; Ferranti, P.; Malorni, A.; et al. Isolation and characterization of four type-1 ribosome-inactivating proteins, with polynucleotide:adenosine glycosidase activity, from leaves of *Phytolacca dioica* L. *Planta* **1999**, *208*, 125–131. [CrossRef]

33. Adwan, H.; Murtaja, A.; Kadhim Al-Taee, K.; Pervaiz, A.; Hielscher, T.; Berger, M.R. Riproximin's activity depends on gene expression and sensitizes PDAC cells to TRAIL. *Cancer Biol. Ther.* **2014**, *15*, 1185–1197. [CrossRef]
34. Ciceroni, C.; Bonelli, M.; Mastrantoni, E.; Niccolini, C.; Laurenza, M.; Larocca, L.M.; Pallini, R.; Traficante, A.; Spinsanti, P.; Ricci-Vitiani, L.; et al. Type-3 metabotropic glutamate receptors regulate chemoresistance in glioma stem cells, and their levels are inversely related to survival in patients with malignant gliomas. *Cell Death Differ.* **2013**, *20*, 396–407. [CrossRef] [PubMed]
35. Surawicz, T.S.; Davis, F.; Freels, S.; Laws, E.R., Jr.; Menck, H.R. Brain tumor survival: Results from the National Cancer Data Base. *J. Neurooncol.* **1998**, *40*, 151–160. [CrossRef] [PubMed]
36. Huszthy, P.C.; Daphu, I.; Niclou, S.P.; Stieber, D.; Nigro, J.M.; Sakariassen, P.O.; Miletic, H.; Thorsen, F.; Bjerkvig, R. In Vivo models of primary brain tumors: Pitfalls and perspectives. *Neuro Oncol.* **2012**, *14*, 979–993. [CrossRef] [PubMed]
37. Mahesparan, R.; Read, T.A.; Lund-Johansen, M.; Skaftnesmo, K.O.; Bjerkvig, R.; Engebraaten, O. Expression of extracellular matrix components in a highly infiltrative in vivo glioma model. *Acta Neuropathol.* **2003**, *105*, 49–57. [CrossRef] [PubMed]
38. Fabbrini, M.S.; Katayama, M.; Nakase, I.; Vago, R. Plant Ribosome-Inactivating Proteins: Progesses, Challenges and Biotechnological Applications (and a Few Digressions). *Toxins* **2017**, *9*, 314. [CrossRef] [PubMed]
39. Rosenblum, M.G.; Cheung, L.H.; Liu, Y.; Marks, J.W., 3rd. Design, expression, purification, and characterization, In Vitro and in vivo, of an antimelanoma single-chain Fv antibody fused to the toxin gelonin. *Cancer Res.* **2003**, *63*, 3995–4002.
40. Shang, C.; Chen, Q.; Dell, A.; Haslam, S.M.; De Vos, W.H.; Van Damme, E.J. The Cytotoxicity of Elderberry Ribosome-Inactivating Proteins Is Not Solely Determined by Their Protein Translation Inhibition Activity. *PLoS ONE* **2015**, *10*, e0132389. [CrossRef]
41. Narayanan, S.; Surendranath, K.; Bora, N.; Surolia, A.; Karande, A.A. Ribosome inactivating proteins and apoptosis. *FEBS Lett.* **2005**, *579*, 1324–1331. [CrossRef]
42. Haar, C.P.; Hebbar, P.; Wallace, G.C.t.; Das, A.; Vandergrift, W.A., 3rd.; Smith, J.A.; Giglio, P.; Patel, S.J.; Ray, S.K.; Banik, N.L. Drug resistance in glioblastoma: A mini review. *Neurochem. Res.* **2012**, *37*, 1192–1200. [CrossRef]
43. Schneider, S.W.; Ludwig, T.; Tatenhorst, L.; Braune, S.; Oberleithner, H.; Senner, V.; Paulus, W. Glioblastoma cells release factors that disrupt blood-brain barrier features. *Acta Neuropathol.* **2004**, *107*, 272–276. [CrossRef]
44. Sarkaria, J.N.; Hu, L.S.; Parney, I.F.; Pafundi, D.H.; Brinkmann, D.H.; Laack, N.N.; Giannini, C.; Burns, T.C.; Kizilbash, S.H.; Laramy, J.K.; et al. Is the blood-brain barrier really disrupted in all glioblastomas? A critical assessment of existing clinical data. *Neuro Oncol.* **2018**, *20*, 184–191. [CrossRef]

toxins

MDPI

Article

DT389-YP7, a Recombinant Immunotoxin against Glypican-3 That Inhibits Hepatocellular Cancer Cells: An In Vitro Study

Hamid Hashemi Yeganeh [1,2], Mohammad Heiat [1], Marek Kieliszek [3], Seyed Moayed Alavian [1] and Ehsan Rezaie [2,*]

[1] Baqiyatallah Research Center for Gastroenterology and Liver Diseases, Baqiyatallah University of Medical Sciences, Tehran 1435916471, Iran; hamid_hashemi001@yahoo.com (H.H.Y.); mohamad.heiat@gmail.com (M.H.); alavian@thc.ir (S.M.A.)

[2] Molecular Biology Research Center, Systems Biology and Poisonings Institute, Baqiyatallah University of Medical Sciences, Tehran 1435916471, Iran

[3] Department of Food Biotechnology and Microbiology, Institute of Food Sciences, Warsaw University of Life Sciences—SGGW, Nowoursynowska 159 C, 02–776 Warsaw, Poland; marek_kieliszek@sggw.edu.pl

* Correspondence: rezaie.ehs@gmail.com; Tel.: +98-21-82454555; Fax: +98-21-83062555

Abstract: Hepatocellular carcinoma (HCC) is one of the high-metastatic types of cancer, and metastasis occurs in one-third of patients with HCC. To maintain the effectiveness of drug compounds on cancer cells and minimize their side effects on normal cells, it is important to use new approaches for overcoming malignancies. Immunotoxins (ITs), an example of such a new approach, are protein-structured compounds consisting of toxic and binding moieties which can specifically bind to cancer cells and efficiently induce cell death. Here, we design and scrutinize a novel immunotoxin against an oncofetal marker on HCC cells. We applied a truncated diphtheria toxin (DT389) without binding domain as a toxin moiety to be fused with a humanized YP7 scFv against a high-expressed Glypican-3 (GPC3) antigen on the surface of HCC cells. Cytotoxic effects of this IT were investigated on HepG2 ($GPC3^+$) and SkBr3 ($GPC3^-$) cell lines as positive- and negative-expressed GPC3 antigens. The dissociation constant (Kd) was calculated 11.39 nM and 18.02 nM for IT and YP7 scfv, respectively, whereas only IT showed toxic effects on the HepG2 cell line, and decreased cell viability (IC50 = 848.2 ng/mL). Changing morphology (up to 85%), cell cycle arrest at G2 phase (up to 13%), increasing intracellular reactive oxygen species (ROSs) (up to 50%), inducing apoptosis (up to 38% for apoptosis and 23% for necrosis), and an almost complete inhibition of cell movement were other effects of immunotoxin treatment on HepG2 cells, not on SkBr3 cell line. These promising results reveal that this new recombinant immunotoxin can be considered as an option as an HCC inhibitor. However, more extensive studies are needed to accomplish this concept.

Keywords: Glypican-3; hepatocellular carcinoma; humanized YP7; diphtheria toxin; new recombinant immunotoxin

Key Contribution: We designed the new diphtheria-based immunotoxin (DT389-YP7) against hepatocellular carcinoma. DT389-YP7 properly inhibits HCC cells by key effects including cell morphology alteration, colony-formation ability impairing, ROS levels elevation, induction of apoptosis, cell cycle arrest and cell movement inhibition. So, this new immunotoxin seems to be a good candidate for pre-clinical studies.

Citation: Hashemi Yeganeh, H.; Heiat, M.; Kieliszek, M.; Alavian, S.M.; Rezaie, E. DT389-YP7, a Recombinant Immunotoxin against Glypican-3 That Inhibits Hepatocellular Cancer Cells: An In Vitro Study. *Toxins* **2021**, *13*, 749. https://doi.org/10.3390/toxins13110749

Received: 22 September 2021
Accepted: 13 October 2021
Published: 22 October 2021

1. Introduction

Out-of-control growth and proliferation of cells lead to tumor formation [1]. Traditional approaches, such as surgery, radiation therapy, chemotherapy, or a combination of them, in treating malignancies are insufficient and accompanied by many side effects on normal tissues [2,3]. Achieving a new technology or tool for cancer-specific treatment is one of the big topics of conversation in medical research [4,5].

The development of anticancer drugs against specific antigens of cancer cells is one of the new attractive methods for researchers to treat cancers [6–8]. As such, in line with this approach, the first, and probably the main, milestone is discovering an appropriated specific antigen as a cancer cell marker [9,10]. GPC3 is a glycophosphatidylinositol (GPI)-anchored cell surface heparan sulfate proteoglycan that is expressed during the early stage of cancer [11], but not in normal adult tissues [12]. GPC3, as an oncofetal antigen, is over-expressed in HCC cells and involved in tumor development through Wnt [13,14], Yap [15], and TGFβ2 [16] signaling pathways. It is detectable on several carcinomas/neoplasms. HCC, yolk sac tumors, thyroid cancer, colorectal carcinoma, gastric carcinoma, pancreatic cancer, and non-small cell lung cancer are the major tissues with GPC3 overexpression. However, evidence has shown that GPC3 is overexpressed in 14% of gastrointestinal tract and pancreatic carcinomas/neoplasms [17]. Meanwhile, HCC with more than 80% expression is taken into account as the most overexpressing tissue [18]. Targeting of such an overexpressed specific antigen on cancer cells by antibodies, or their derivatives, is tempting as an efficient strategy to annihilate cancer cells [19–21]. ITs are protein structures consisting of two parts: the toxin and the binding moieties. Herbal or bacterial toxins can be used as a toxin moiety in the structure of ITs. As such, the potent toxins are raised as key agents in cancer treatment, as well as in protection against infectious agents [22]. The binding moiety contains a specific monoclonal antibody or binding fragment, such as the antigen-binding (Fab) or the single-chain fragment variable (scFv) [23,24]. Specific binding of the antibody to the antigen causes the toxin to enter into the cancer cells, subsequently killing the cell by inhibiting protein synthesis. This specific binding diminishes the negative effects of immunotoxins on normal cells [25].

Multiple ITs have been designed against GPC3 of hepatocellular cancer cells [26,27]. One of the problems associated with antibody-based therapies is the secondary immune response to animal-derived therapeutic antibodies as foreign antigens. To overcome this problem, humanized antibodies have been developed in which complementarity-determining regions (CDRs) of the antibody remain intact, and other regions are substituted with their counterparts in human antibodies [28]. Other than humanization, reducing the size of the antibodies can also decrease the secondary immune responses. The functional fragments of antibodies, such as scFvs, nanobodies, and Fab fragments, are much considered in this regard. Yi-Fan Zhang et al. investigated and compered several humanized scFv against GPC3, and provided us with a clear picture of the biological and physicochemical status of existing structures [28]. On the other hand, choosing a meet toxin is another challenge in designing and manufacturing of ITs. The size, function, toxicity, and immunogenicity of the toxin moiety are the bottlenecks for selecting an appropriate toxin.

Summarizing these issues in a valid concept calls for the conduction of a study with the aim of designing and producing an engineered IT structure, and evaluating its bioactivities. Accordingly, after in-silico analysis on different IT constructions composed of previously developed scFvs [28], a truncated diphtheria toxin, and different number of linkers, the best-scored structure was chosen to be produced, and its effect on HCC cells investigated. As such, after the expression and purification of the recombinant IT, its binding affinity and cell toxicity on HepG2 as a hepatocellular carcinoma cell line were investigated.

2. Results

2.1. Construction Design

Although in-silico analysis and physic-chemical properties of the three structures were the same, the DT389-$(GGGGS)_2$-YP7 IT showed more reliable conformation and structural orientation (Figure 1a). After codon adaptation of DT389-$(GGGGS)_2$-YP7 IT based on the *E. coli* strand, the primary expression was optimized and prepared for continued investigation.

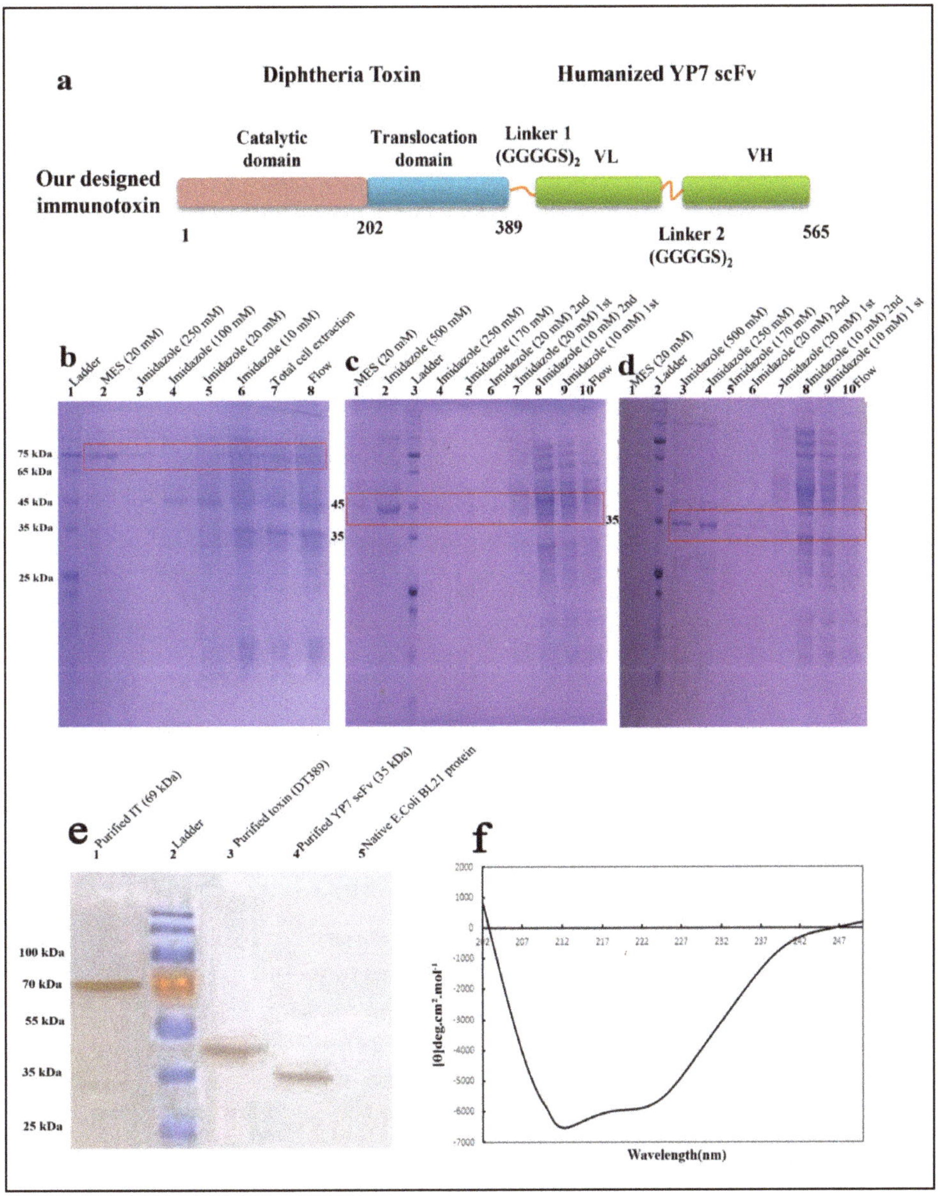

Figure 1. Schematic structures of DT389-(GGGGS)$_2$-YP7 immunotoxin. The truncated *Diphtheria* (DT389) was fused to humanized YP7 scFv (developed byY. Zhang et al., 2016) against GPC3 antigen, by two repeats of G_4S flexible linker (**a**). Purification and validation of proteins using Ni-NTA column and western blotting. Conformational and secondary structure study of IT through CD analysis. Purification of DT389-(GGGGS)2-YP7 IT (**b**), DT389, and humanized YP7 scFv was performed using affinity chromatography and different concentrations of imidazole to achieve the most purified protein of interest on 12% SDS-PAGE. (**b**). 1: ladder, 2: elution buffer containing MES (20 mM), 3: elution buffer containing 250 mM imidazole, 4: elution buffer containing 100 mM imidazole, 5: washing buffer containing 20 mM imidazole, 6: washing buffer containing 10 mM imidazole, 7: total sonicated cell extraction, 8: flow through from column. (**c**). 1: elution buffer containing MES (20 mM), 2: elution buffer containing 500 mM imidazole, 3: ladder, 4: elution buffer containing 250 mM imidazole, 5: elution buffer containing 170 mM imidazole, 6: second washing buffer containing 20 mM imidazole, 7: first washing buffer

containing 20 mM imidazole, 8: second washing buffer containing 10 mM imidazole, 9: first washing buffer containing 10 mM imidazole, 10: flow through from column. (**d**). 1: elution buffer containing MES (20 mM), 2: ladder, 3: elution buffer containing 500 mM imidazole, 4: elution buffer containing 250 mM imidazole, 5: elution buffer containing 170 mM imidazole, 6: second washing buffer containing 20 mM imidazole, 7: first washing buffer containing 20 mM imidazole, 8: second washing buffer containing 10 mM imidazole, 9: first washing buffer containing 10 mM imidazole, 10: flow through from column. (**e**). Validating of proteins were performed by western blotting. Results showed that purification of proteins was accurate. 1: purified IT (69 kDa), 2: ladder, 3: purified truncated Diphtheria (DT389) (42 kDa), 4: purified YP7 scFv (35 kDa), 5: total protein extraction of native *E. coli* BL21 without vector. (**f**). Secondary structure of IT using far-CD. Main percentage of secondary structure was dedicated to be α-Helix.

2.2. *Purification and Validation of Proteins*

Purified proteins were analyzed by SDS-PAGE and western blotting (Figure 1a–c). The same purification protocol, as mentioned above, was followed for all three proteins. The most purified protein fraction was eluted in higher concentrations of imidazole (500 mM) and MES (20 mg/mL) buffers. A single band on 12% SDS-Page gel indicated purified proteins. Purification process was carried out separately for DT389-$(GGGGS)_2$-YP7 IT (Figure 2b), DT389 (Figure 2c), and humanized YP7 scFv (Figure 2d). To validate purified proteins, the recombinant proteins were detected by Anti His-Tag antibodies and western blot analysis (Figure 2e). Three single bands in 69, 42, and 35 kDa were related to purified IT, truncated *Diphtheria* (DT389), and humanized YP7 scFv, respectively.

The data from conformational analysis indicated that the expression and purification processes have been performed correctly, and SDS-PAGE visualized bands were dedicated to our interested proteins.

Using the GOR IV online server, the secondary structure of IT (DT389-$(GGGGS)_2$-YP7) was predicted and compered to experimental data obtained from far-CD (Figure 1f). Experimental analysis on IT structure showed more α-helix and extended strand structures than the in silico predicted structure (Table 1). The percentage of α-helix, extended strand, and random coil in the experimental model were calculated as 40.23%, 29.81%, and 29.96%, respectively. Among these, the percentages of alpha helix and extended strand are slightly more than predicted percentages.

2.3. *Binding Affinity and Bioactivity*

Binding of IT, DT389, and YP7 scFv to HepG2 and SkBr3 cell lines was investigated by cell-ELISA. Results revealed that IT and YP7 scFv bind to HepG2 cells, whereas DT389 could not. The Kd of IT and YP7 scFv was 11.38 nM and 18.02 nM, respectively, on HepG2 ($GPC3^+$) cells (Figure 2a). SkBr3 (GPC3) cells as negative control showed no binding attachment for IT, DT389, and YP7 scFv (Figure 2b).

The viability of HepG2 cells was decreased by increasing of IT concentration with an IC50 value of 848.2 ng/mL (Figure 2c), whereas no toxic effect was detected on SkBr3 (Figure 2d). Neither DT389 nor YP7 scFv had a toxic effect on either type of the cancer cell lines. The number of cell death induced by IT, DT389, and YP7 scFv was investigated by trypan blue staining. The results demonstrated that when increasing the concentration of IT, the number of HepG2 dead cells would also be increased (Figure 2e).

2.4. *Cells' Morphology*

The morphology of HepG2 cells altered after treatment with IT (Figure 3a). Increasing the concentration of IT resulted in a decrease in the number of cells, colony-forming ability, size of cells, and adherent property. In high concentrations (≥1000 ng/mL), cell shrinkage and decreasing cell asymmetry shape were occurred. Acridine orange/ethidium bromide staining of HepG2 cells revealed that IT (850 and 1250 ng/mL) induces apoptosis. Cell membrane lobulation and DNA fragmentation was observed in IT-treated HepG2 cells. All of the SkBr3 cells were intact even in the presence of the highest concentration of IT (Figure 3b). As the results show, DT389 and scFv had no effect on both HepG2 and SkBr3 cell lines.

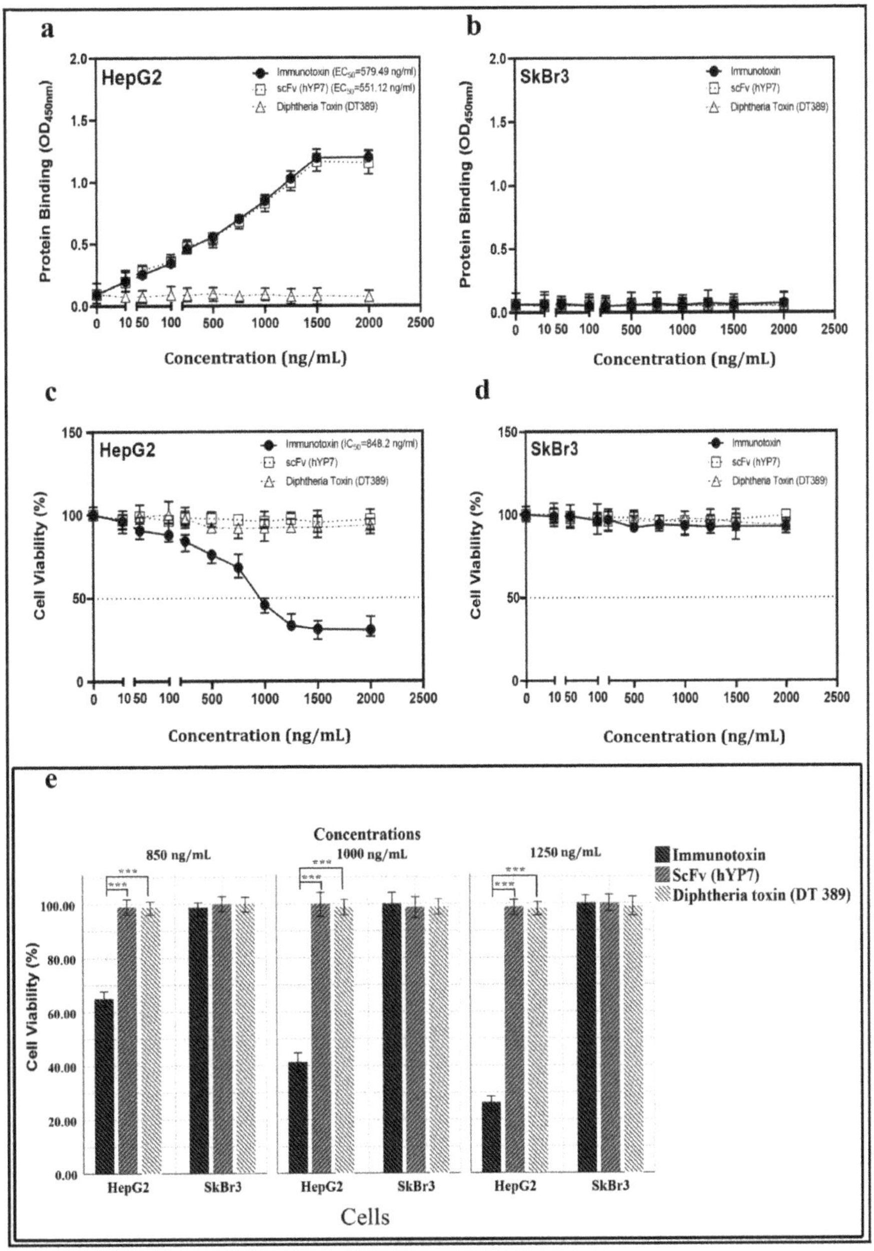

Figure 2. Investigation of binding affinity (**a**,**b**) and toxicity (**e**) of IT, DT389, and YP7 scFv proteins on HepG2 and SkBr3 cell lines after 24 h of treatment. The Kd of immunotoxin, DT389, and YP7 scFv to HepG2 (**a**) and SkBr3 cells (**b**) with different concentrations of each three proteins separately (0, 50, 100, 250, 500, 750, 1000, 1250, 1500, and 2000 ng/mL) using cell-ELISA approach. OD450 nm represented as binding property. Toxic effect of IT, DT389, and YP7 scF on HepG2 cells (**c**) and SkBr3 cells (**d**) with the same concentrations using MTT assay. Decreasing cell viability was observed at higher concentrations of immunotoxin (≥1000 ng/mL) in HepG2 cells. (**e**) Trypan blue assay was used to confirm cell toxicity of immunotoxin. Number of blue-colored cells represented as dead cells in comparison with control group. Results were expressed as the mean ± SD. (*** $p < 0.001$) ($n = 3$).

Table 1. Result of secondary structure obtained from fat CD.

Type of Fusion Protein	Alpha Helix	Extended Strand	Random Coil
DT289-(GGGGS)2-YP7	40.23	29.81	29.96

The analyzed data are displayed in percentage.

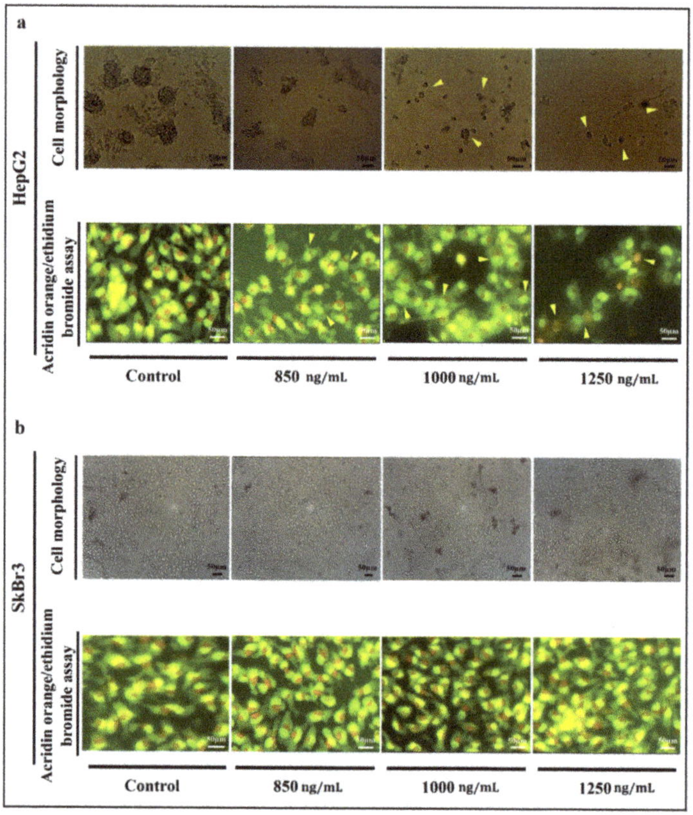

Figure 3. Morphology of HpG2 (**a**) and SkBr3 cell lines (**b**) investigation using optical and fluorescent microscopes. (**a**) Morphology of HepG2 cells was changed after treatment with IT. A decrease in the number of cells and colony-forming ability, cell membrane destruction, and cell shrinkage were observed as main changes (marked cell). Acridine-orange ethidium bromide staining revealed that the rate of apoptosis (early and late) and necrosis were raised up at highest concentrations (1250 ng/mL) of IT compared to control. Cell membrane lobulation and DNA fragmentation were observed in lower concentration of IT (≤1000 ng/mL). (**b**) The same concentrations of IT were applied to SkBr3 cell line, however, no morphologic changes were observed after treatment.

2.5. Apoptosis and Cell Cycle

New recombinant IT activated an apoptosis pathway in HepG2 cells. Twenty-four hours after treatments, HepG2 cells migrated to an apoptosis area division, and the percentage of living normal cell decreased undergoing IT treatment, whereas no decrease of living normal cells in the SkBr3 cell line was observed. The percentage of early and late apoptosis, and necrotic cells, increased compared to control in HepG2 cells when increasing IT concentration (20.2 and 4.49% for early apoptosis, 14.8 and 34.0% for late apoptosis, and

2.63 and 23.0% for necrotic cells were observed after treatment of cells with 850 and 1250 ng/mL of IT, respectively) (Figure 4).

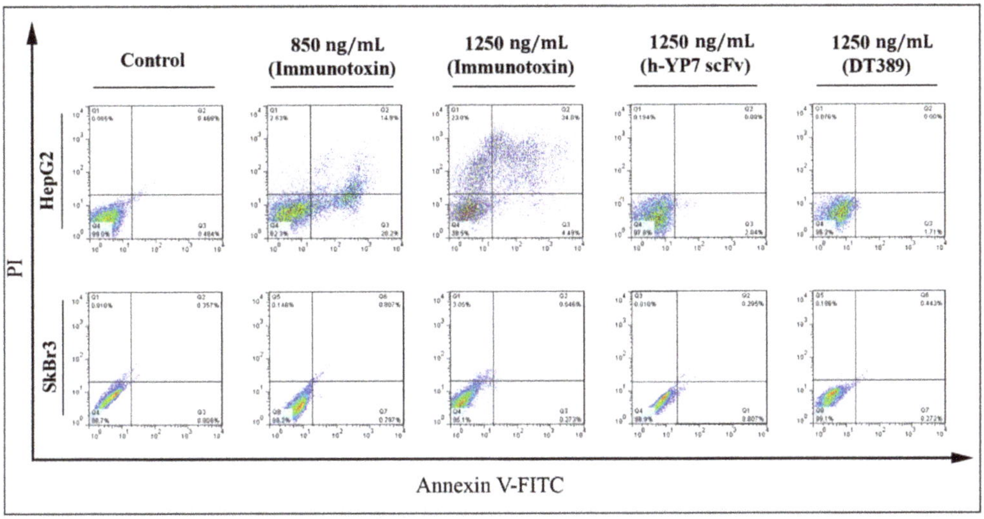

Figure 4. Effect of IT, DT389, and YP7 scFv on apoptosis induction after 24 of treatment using flow cytometry. Categorization of treated cells into necrotic cells (Q1), late apoptosis (Q2), early apoptosis (Q3), and normal cells (Q4). After treatment, HepG2 cells moved into apoptosis and then, necrosis regions. Results were analyzed by FlowJo software. Data have been shown for a single sample.

Reactive oxygen species (ROSs) in the cells were increased under treatment with IT. ROS participated in the oxidative pathway and consequently, cell death. Increasing dichlorofluorescein (DCF) represented as internal ROS in cells, which is detectable by flow cytometry. By increasing the concentration of IT, the emission intensity in HepG2 cells was increased (Figure 5a), so that 7.1% of pretreatment HepG2 cells with positive internal ROS increased significantly to 39.7% and 57.5% in treated cells with 850 and 1250 ng/mL of IT, respectively (Figure 5b).

HepG2 cell cycle arrest was also observed under treatment with IT. Based on the intensity of PI staining, cells divided to sub-G1, G1, S, and G2 phases (Figure 6a). The percentage of cells at sub-G1 was increased from 2.89% in the HepG2 control cell line to 10.3% and 16.9% after treatment with 850 and 1250 ng/mL of IT, respectively (Figure 6b). Cells arrest at the G2 phase, and an increase of ROS resulted in more cell apoptosis induction. No cellular effect (neither HepG2 nor SkBr3 cell lines) was observed after treatment with DT389 and YP7 scFv, which indicated that none of them had the capability to inhibit cancer cells on their own.

2.6. Cell Movement and Metastasis

Movement of HepG2 cells was prevented after IT treatment. Inhibition of cell movement was investigated using scratch and cell invasion assays. Compared to control, higher concentrations of IT ($\geq$1000 ng/mL) caused the related distance of edges to remain intact, and had no inhibitory effect on SkBr3 cells (Figure 7a). The average distance from edges to edge of cell was measured and considered as cell movement. Statistical analysis indicated a significant difference between treated target cells and related controls (Figure 7b).

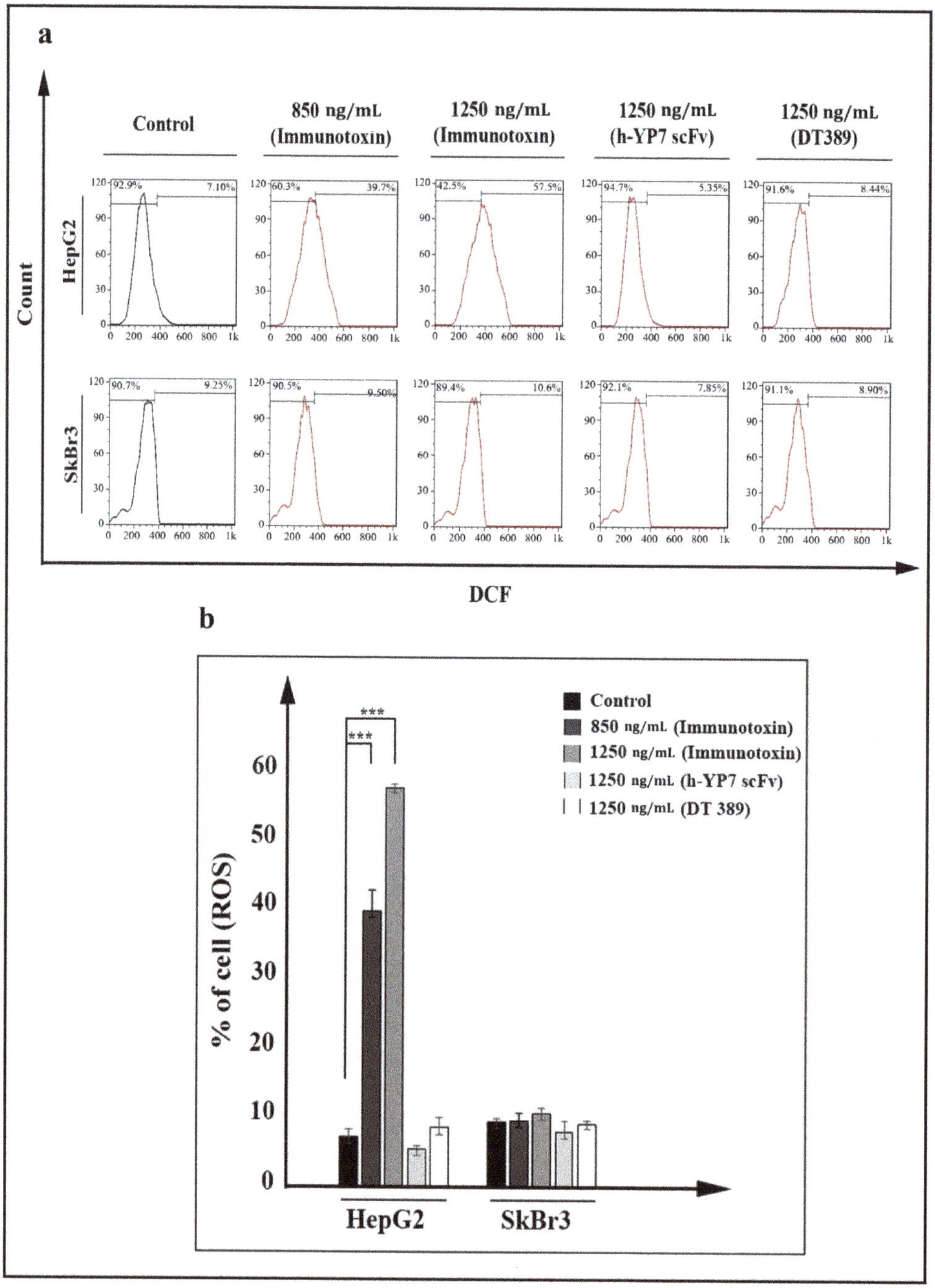

Figure 5. Reactive oxygen species (ROSs) increasing in HepG2 cells treated by IT after 24 h. (**a**) Increasing fluorescent DCF, represented as intracellular ROS in IT treated HepG2 cells (data have been shown for a single sample). (**b**) Percentage of ROS-positive cells was meanly increased at 850 and 1250 ng/mL concentrations of IT in HepG2 cells. Results were analyzed by FlowJo software and expressed as the mean ± SD. (*** $p < 0.001$) ($n = 3$).

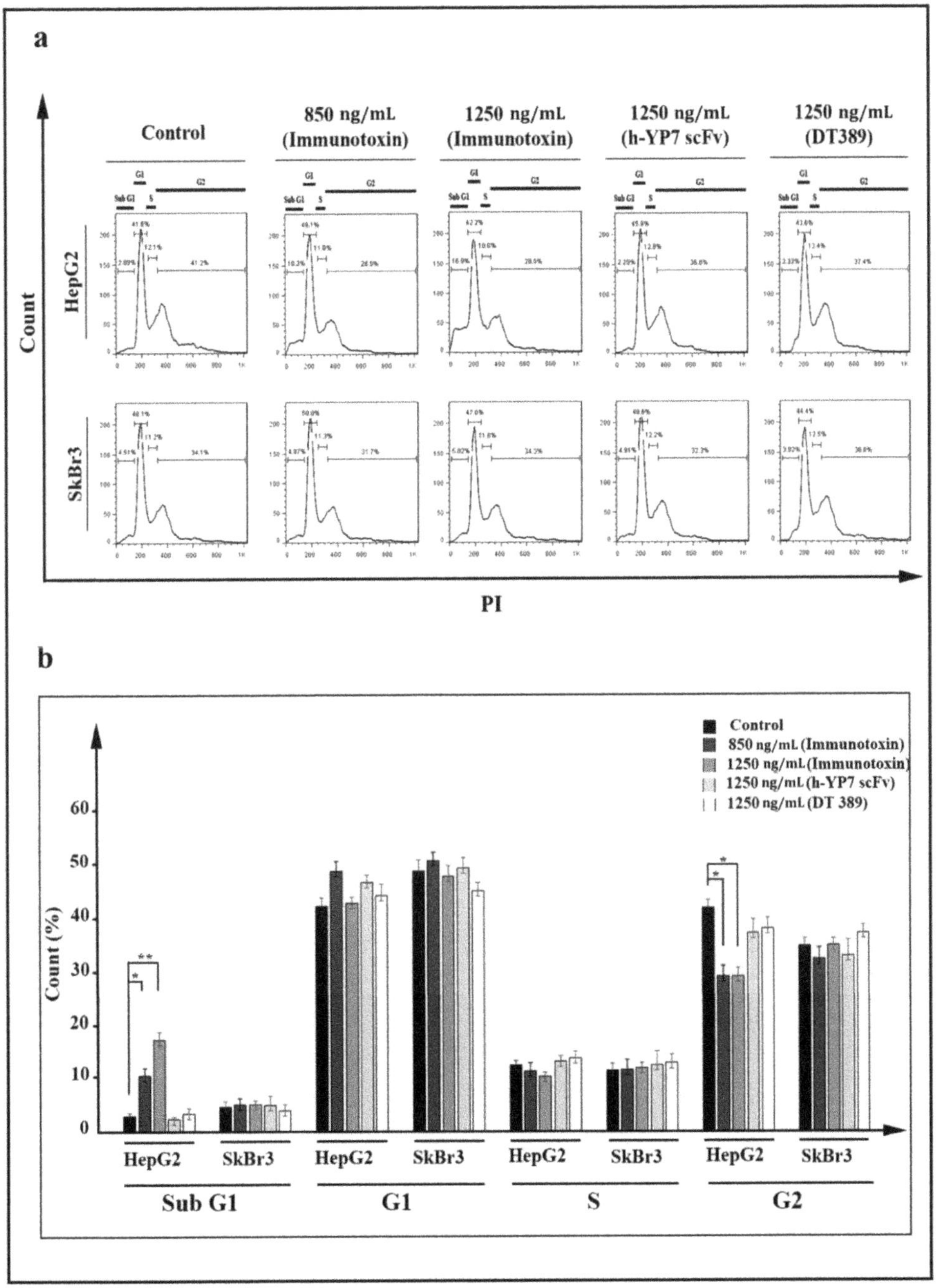

Figure 6. Cell cycle arrest following IT-treatment of HepG2 cells after 24 h. (**a**) Cell cycle was arrested in HepG2 cells treated with IT at G2 phase, but not in SkBr3 cells. Propidium iodide (PI) dye was utilized to stain DNA strands. Different amounts of DNA (single or double strand) were considered to distinguish cells (data have been shown for a single sample). (**b**) Percentage of cells in different phases sub-G1, G1, S, and G2. Distribution of cells in sub-G1 phase increased after IT treatment in HepG2 cells. Results were analyzed by FlowJo software and expressed as the mean ± SD. (* $p < 0.05$ and ** $p < 0.01$) ($n = 3$).

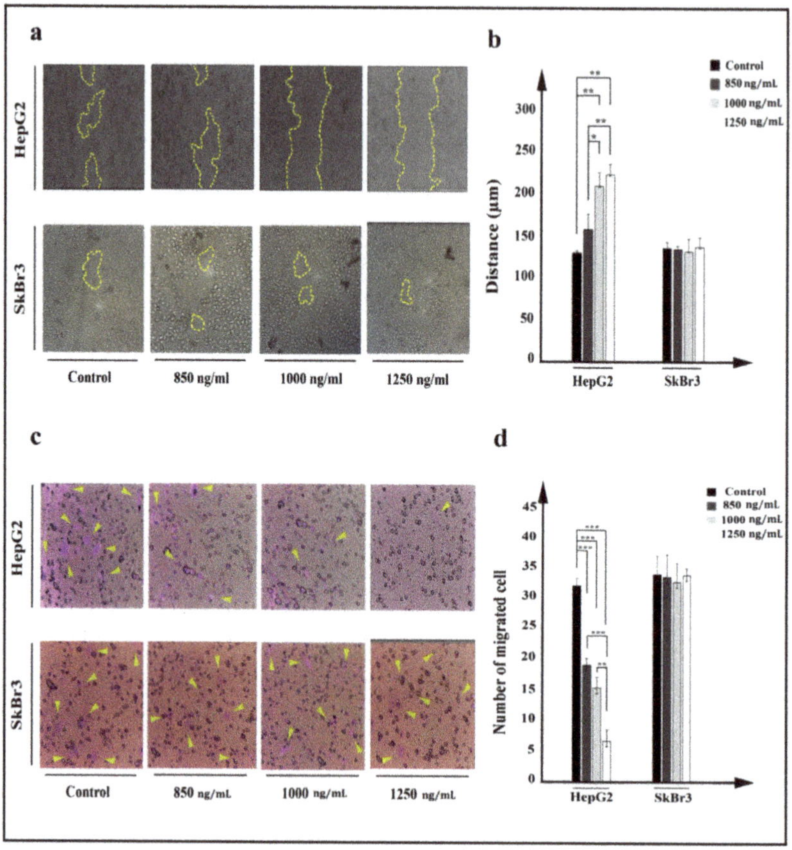

Figure 7. Investigation of effect of IT on HepG2 (**a**,**b**) and SkBr3 cell movement after 24 h treatment with 850, 1000, and 1250 ng/mL of IT. (**a**). Movement of HepG2 and SkBr3 cells was inhibited after treatment. (**b**). Average of distances between edge to edge was measured using ImageJ software, and data were presented as the mean (µm) ± SD. (**c**). After 24 h of migration, passed cells through pores were stained by crystal violet and counted using a fluorescence microscope. (**d**). Passed cells were counted and compared to control in both HepG2 and SkBr3 cell lines. Results were expressed as the mean ± SD. (* $p < 0.05$, ** $p < 0.01$, and *** $p < 0.001$) ($n = 3$).

Cancer cells' property to change the cytoskeleton and move throughout pores was investigated by a cell invasion assay. A plate with a chamber covered by 8 µm diameter pores was utilized to evaluate property of IT-treated cell to cross through pores, in which passed cells were considered as metastatic cells. The number of passed HepG2 cells was significantly decreased after treatment with IT (Figure 7c). Higher concentrations of IT (≥1000 ng/mL) were more effective in inhibiting cells movement, and in the HepG2 cell line, 32 passed cells in control decreased to 20, 12, and 6 cells at 850, 1000, and 1250 ng/mL concentrations of IT, respectively. No effect was seen on SkBr3 cell line (Figure 7d).

3. Discussion

Since 2000, many ITs have been designed to inhibit hepatocellular carcinoma (HCC) cells [29,30]. The variety in scFv and toxin moieties has caused various ITs with different binding affinities and IC50 [14,26,27,31,32].

Pseudomonas exotoxin A (PE), as one of the prominent toxin moieties, is mostly used in IT structures. The intrinsic properties of PE, including, high toxicity, well-known routing and processing, and ease of manipulation, have given it some superiorities over other toxin moieties [33]. PE, possessing the furin cleavable and KDEL-like motifs, facilitates further detaching of the catalytic domain and retrograde transportation to the endoplasmic reticulum (ER), respectively [34].

Diphtheria toxin (DT) is another successful toxin moiety in which the R-domain is substituted with a targeting moiety to construct ITs. DT, like PE, has a furin cleavable moiety, and functionally has shown low IC50. ONTAK, as the only FDA approved IT (certified in 1999), is a DT-based IT against cutaneous T-cell lymphoma.

The other arm of IT is a targeting moiety. To choose the best targeting moiety, it is essential to find a fit target. Evidence has revealed that CPC3 would be an ideal antigen to be used as an IT target in HCCcells. Hitherto, multiple ITs (e.g., HN3, HS20, and YP7) have been introduced against GPC3 [12,16–18]. GPC3 is related to the Yap and Wnt signaling pathways. Findings have demonstrated that HN3 and HS20 have inhibitory effects on both pathways. However, YP7 (a mouse mAb which identified the C-terminal of GPC3) has shown no effect on neither Wnt nor Yap signaling pathways. Nevertheless, all of them have shown anti-tumor activity in vivo [14].

In the present study, several IT structures were designed based on in silico analysis. Among all, the DT389-(GGGGS)$_2$-YP7 immunotoxin was chosen as the main structure, and its structural stability was studied in our laboratory. Considered IT and its components (DT389 and YP7 scFv) were expressed and purified separately using immobilized metal affinity chromatography (IMAC). Western blot and far-CD analyses were performed to confirm accuracy of purified protein and the secondary structure. The Kd for IT and YP7 scFv was 11.39 nM and 18.02 nM, respectively, and IC50 for IT on HepG2 cells was 848.2 ng/mL. No binding affinity for DT389 was observed neither for HepG2 nor SkBr3 cell lines. Besides, DT389 and YP7 scFv showed no cytotoxic effect on HepG2 and SkBr3 cell lines. A lethal effect of IT on the HepG2 cell line was significantly manifested, and at higher concentrations of IT ($\geq$1000 ng/mL), the morphology and colony forming ability of cells were disrupted (Figure 3a).

Previously, the cytotoxic effect of YP7-based immunotoxins has been approved by Zhang and their colleagues, and they designed humanized anti-GPC3 scFvs, namely hYP7 and hYP9.1 fused with PE, and investigated their affinity and cytotoxicity. They grafted the combined KABAT/IMGT complementarity determining regions (CDRs) of mouse scFvs into a human IgG germline framework. In spite of a very similar scFv sequence of mouse YP7-, YP8-, YP9-, and YP9.1-PE38 immunotoxins, the two YP7-PE38 and YP9.1-PE38 showed higher efficiency and performance and subsequently, were chosen to be humanized. In humanized immunotoxins, the binding affinity of hYP9.1-PE38 was better, but hYP7-PE38 was more cytotoxic [28].

DNA fragmentation, as the major feature of early apoptosis cells [35], was observed in HepG2 cells treated with IT. At 1250 ng/mL concentration of IT, the HepG2 cell was promoted to activate the necrosis pathway, as well as the apoptosis pathway. Flow cytometry data analysis also indicated the apoptosis activation and necrosis development in HepG2 cells, but not in SkBr3 cell line.

Protein synthesis inhibition following inactivation of elongation factor 2 (EF2) by the immunotoxin is associated with loss of mitochondrial membrane potential (MtMP), and promotes cells death. Furthermore, it has been revealed that IT induces apoptotic proteins such as Bax and DNA fragmentation factors, cytochrome c (Cyt c) release, and ultimately, caspase-dependent cell death [36–38].

As shown, reactive oxygen species (ROSs) were increased in IT-treated HepG2 cells. It has been demonstrated that ROSs were increased in cancer cells treated with IT through inhibition of antioxidant pathways, such as the KEAP1-NRF2 pathway [39]. In the following, ROSs with their extremely reactive and toxic properties, can oxidize cellular components, and have synergetic effects on cell destruction and death. [40,41].

Data of cell cycle analysis obtained from flow cytometry revealed that our recombinant IT arrests the HepG2 cell cycle at the G2 phase. Previous studies have been shown that ITs can impress cell cycles at G1/S phases [42–44]. Correlation among DNA fragmentation, apoptosis, and cell cycle arrest has been extensively investigated. Increasing Bax as an apoptotic factor represented a transcriptional factor for p53, which is considered a tumor suppressor by inducing cell cycle arrest and cell apoptosis [30,45,46]. Generally, in addition to direct effect of IT on the activation cell apoptosis, increasing intracellular ROS and arresting cells into the G2 phase will confer it the maximum toxic effects.

Metastasis of primary cancer cells to other organs makes cancer cells difficult to cure, so inhibition of cell movement would be a promising way to overcome the challenges of metastatic cancers [47]. Results of a scratch assay and cell invasion assay revealed that the treatment of HepG2 cells with IT reduces the cell movement and invasion (Figure 5). Reducing proteins that participate in cell movement and metastasis is considered a consequence of protein synthesis inhibition followed by IT treatment [48]. As is mentioned above, YP7 is not able to block signaling pathways through binding to GPC3 [14]. As such, it could be reasonable that the reduced movement can only be attributed to cell death. However, more investigations are needed to reach a perfect concept in this regard.

4. Conclusions

In conclusion, DT389-(GGGGS)$_2$-YP7 recombinant IT demonstrated a toxic effect on the HepG2 cell line. Cell morphology alteration, colony-formation ability impairing, ROS levels elevation, induction of apoptosis and cell cycle arrest and cell movement, and metastasis inhibition were the major effects of IT treatment. DT389-(GGGGS)$_2$-YP7 immunotoxin could be considered as a novel recombinant protein to inhibit HCC cells with high expressions of GPC3. However, this underling scientific effort calls for further studies to respond to all questions around this recombinant protein.

5. Materials and Methods

5.1. Construction Design

A variety of structures of ITs were constructed, composed of a truncated diphtheria toxin (residues 1-389; DT389) (Expasy accession no. P00588) [49] and different Yi-Fan Zhang's humanized anti-GPC3 scFvs (YP7, YP8, YP9 and YP9.1) [28], using credible in-silico software. This preliminary phase of studies focused on investigating the effectiveness of different G$_4$S linkers between toxin and scFv moieties on secondary and three-dimensional structures, stability, flexibility, solubility, and physic-chemical properties. In the end, the structure with the highest score (DT389-(GGGGS)$_2$-YP7) was selected as best IT candidate. The nucleotide sequence of the selected construct was synthesized in PET 21a+ and transformed to the *Escherichia coli* strain for recombinant expression. Apart from IT, the toxin and YP7 scFv moieties were separately produced for further analysis. Two- and three-dimensional structure analysis, as well as the degree of stability in all recombinant proteins was investigated.

5.2. Production, Purification, and Validation of Recombinant Protein by Affinity Chromatography and Western Blotting

IT (DT389-(GGGGS)$_2$-YP7), truncated diphtheria (DT389), and scFv (humanized YP7) were produced (under the induction condition of 1 mM isopropyl β-D-1-thiogalactopyranoside (IPTG) at 37 °C for 6 h incubation) and purified using a nickel-nitrilotriacetic acid (Ni–NTA) affinity column. Buffers containing 10, 20, 100, 170, 250, and 500 mM of imidazole and MES (2-(*N*-morpholino) ethane sulfonic acid) buffer were utilized for column calibration, washing, and elution. All eluted fractions were collected separately and analyzed by 12% sodium dodecyl sulfate polyacrylamide gel electrophoresis (SDS-PAGE). The concentrations of recombinant proteins were obtained using a Bradford assay. The purified recombinant proteins were validated by western blotting, and the three proteins were applied to the separate wells of SDS-PAGE. Then, proteins were transferred to a nitrocellulose membrane and blocked with tris-buffered saline (TBS) containing 0.05% Tween 20 (TBST) and 5% skim milk for 2 h in a shaker (SPEED rpm) at room temperature. After removing the blocking buffer and washing with PBST, the nitrocellulose membrane was incubated overnight at 4 °C with 1:2000 diluted horseradish peroxidase (7)-conjugated Anti His-Tag antibodies (Sigma, Berlin, Germany). The membrane was washed three times with TBST, and DAB (3,3′-Diaminobenzidine) substrate was added to detect the proteins of interest.

5.3. *Circular Dichroism Analysis*

The secondary structures (alpha-helix, beta-sheet, beta-turn, or some other conformations (e.g., random coil)) of recombinant proteins were determined by a ultraviolet circular dichroism (CD) spectrum. To do this, the purified proteins (0.3 mg/mL) in buffer were used, and analyzed by a CD spectrum at 180 to 240 nm.

5.4. *Cell Lines and Culture*

Human HepG2 ($GPC3^+$) hepatocellular carcinoma (HCC) and human SkBr3 ($GPC3^-$) breast cancer cell lines were obtained from the cell bank department of Pasture institute (Tehran, Iran), and cultured in supplemented Roswell Park Memorial Institute (RPMI-1640) medium (Gibco, Carlsbad, CA, USA) at 37 °C in 5% CO_2 incubation condition. The media had been supplemented with 10% fetal bovine serum (FBS) (Gibco, CA, USA), and 1% antibiotic (50 U/mL of penicillin and 50 µg/mL streptomycin).

5.5. *Cytotoxic Effect of Immunotoxin*

An MTT assay was performed to investigate the cytotoxic effect of the immunotoxin. HepG2 and SkBr3 cell lines were seeded into the wells of a 96-well plate at a density of 15,000 cells in 200 µL culture medium. After overnight incubation at 37 °C in 5% CO_2, cells were separately exposed with different concentrations (10, 50, 100, 250, 500, 750, 1000, 1250, 1500, 2000 ng/mL) of DT389-$(GGGGS)_2$-YP7 immunotoxin, DT389, and humanized scFv (YP7). Then, cells were incubated at 37 °C for 24 h. Thereafter, 30 µL of 3-(4,5-dimethylthiazol-2-yl)-2,5-diphenyltetrazolium bromide (MTT) stock solution (5 mg/mL) was added into each well, and the incubation was continued for 4 h. Afterward, dimethyl sulfoxide (DMSO) was added to dissolved formed formazan crystals by living cells. Subsequently, the absorbance of the solution was measured at 570 nm by an ELISA microplate reader (Spectra MAX Plus; Molecular Devices, San Jose, CA, USA).

A trypan blue assay was also used to determine the immunotoxin-mediated cell death. After 24 h of cell treatments with 850, 1000, and 1250 ng/mL of each immunotoxin, DT389, or YP7 scFv proteins, cells were harvested and mixed with a trypan blue stain [1;1], and counted using a hemocytometer and inverted microscope (Nikon Instruments Inc., Tokyo, Japan). Blue cells were considered as death cells.

5.6. *Cell Morphology Analysis*

To investigate the morphology of cells, 120,000 cells/well were seeded in a 12-well plate and after treatment with different concentrations of immunotoxin (850, 1000, and 1250 ng/mL), the cell morphology was analyzed using an inverted microscope. Acridine orange/ethidium bromide staining of treated cells was carried out to detect apoptotic and necrotic cells. An amount of 250 µL/well of acridin orange and ethidium bromide (24 mg/mL for both of them) was added to cells and incubated for 3 min. Cells were washed twice with PBS (1×) and analyzed using fluorescence microscopy.

5.7. *Cell Enzyme-Linked Immunosorbent Assay (Cell-ELISA)*

A cell-ELISA test was used to investigate the affinity binding of recombinant proteins to $GPC3^+$ cells. In this regard, 15,000 cells/wells were seeded into microtiter plates (Nunc-ImmunoPlates® Maxisorp, Frankfurt, Germany) and incubated at 37 °C upon reaching 70% confluence. After cell fixation by formaldehyde (10% *v*/*v*) and blocking with PBS-BSA solution (6% *w*/*v*), the cells were treated with different concentrations of DT389-$(GGGGS)_2$-YP7 immunotoxin, DT389, and humanized YP7 scFv, as mentioned in the MTT assay. After washing with PBST four times (PBS (1×) containing 0.05% Tween-20), the diluted

Anti-His Tag antibodies (1:16,000 in PBST) were added into each well. The plates were then incubated for 60 min at 37 °C. Thereafter, each well was washed four times with PBST to remove non-specific antibodies. Finally, 3,3′,5,5′-tetramethylbenzidine (TMB-H_2O_2; Sigma-Aldrich, St. Louis, MO, USA) solution was added, and color development proceeded for 20 min before the addition of a stop solution (2 M H_2SO_4). The absorbance value of each well was measured at 450 nm using a microplate reader (Bio-Rad, Hercules, CA, USA). The resulting data were expressed in terms of OD values.

5.8. Annexin V/PI Apoptosis Detection

Apoptotic effects of recombinant proteins were investigated on HepG2 and ShBr3 cells using an Annexin V/propidium iodide (PI) assay. Cells were seeded into a 12-well plate incubated at 37 °C to reach 60% related confluence. Cells were treated with different concentrations of immunotoxin (850 and 1250 ng/mL), DT389 (1250 ng/mL), and YP7 scFv (1250 ng/mL), and incubated at 37 °C for 24 h. Cells were harvested and washed twice with PBS (1×), and resuspended in binding buffer. Categorization of cells into four horizons, including alive, early and late apoptotic, and necrotic cells, was determined by an Annexin V/PI staining kite. Fluorescein isothiocyanate (FITC)–conjugated Annexin V/PI solution was added and incubated at room temperature for 30 min. Apoptosis analysis was carried out using FACSCalibur™ Flow Cytometer (BD Biosciences, San Jose, CA, USA).

5.9. Cell Cycle Investigation

Analysis of cell distribution in different phases of cell cycle (subG1, G1, S, and G2) was performed using PI staining and a flow cytometric assay. After treatment of cells with concentrations of immunotoxin (850 and 1250 ng/mL), DT389 (1250 ng/mL), and YP7 scFv (1250 ng/mL) defined for 24 h, cells were harvested and fixed with ethanol 70% (*v*/*v*) for 30 min. Then, the cells were washed twice with PBS (1×) and propidium iodide (10 μg/mL) was added to determine cell distribution using a FACSCalibur™ Flow Cytometer. Results were analyzed by FlowJo™ Software version 7.6.1.

5.10. Quantification of ROS in Cells

Dichloro-dihydro-fluorescein diacetate (DCFH-DA) passes through cell membrane, and is oxidated to convert to fluorescent molecule dichlorofluorescein (DCF) by reactive oxygen species (ROSs). To perform this test, the same cell counts were seeded and treated as cell cycle analysis. Treated cells were incubated with 10 μM of DCFH-DA for 1 h. The emission fluorescent was measured using a flow cytometer, and its data were analyzed by FlowJo software version 7.6.1.

5.11. Cell Migration

Migration of cells was investigated using scratch and cell invasion assays. For the scratch assay, a 12-well plate was coated by cells overnight and then treated with 850, 1000, and 1250 ng/mL of immunotoxin. A central cell-free line was created using a sterile yellow tip, and cells were permitted to migrate for the next 24 h. Distance between scratch edges was calculated using ImageJ 1.48 software.

The cell invasion assay was performed using a Transwell™ plate with a special chamber containing 8 μm diameter pores at the bottom. After treatment of cells with 850, 1000, and 1250 ng/mL concentration of immunotoxin for 24 h, 10,000 treated cells of each concentration were added into the upper chamber containing 100 μL cell culture medium with 2% FBS. In the lower part, cell culture medium with 10% FBS was added, and cells were permitted to move through pores for 48 h. Passed cells were fixed using ethanol 70% (*v*/*v*), and stained with 0.1% (*w*/*v*) crystal violet for 5 min. Stained cells were investigated using an inverted microscope. The process of cell migration was explored by inverted microscope visualization.

5.12. Statistical Analyses

Data were presented as means ± standard deviations. All experiments were repeated in triplicate. Using IBM SPSS statistics 26, all data were analyzed. Significant statistical differences among the groups, obtained from fit statistical tests, are presented with * $p < 0.05$, ** $p < 0.01$, and *** $p < 0.001$ in histograms.

Author Contributions: Conceptualization, E.R. and M.H.; writing—original draft preparation H.H.Y. and E.R.; writing—review and editing, M.K., S.M.A., M.H. and E.R.; visualization, M.K., S.M.A. and M.H.; validation, E.R.; Funding acquisition, S.M.A.; supervision, E.R. All authors have read and agreed to the published version of the manuscript.

Funding: This work was supported by the NIMAD: National institute for medical research development under grant number 983134.

Institutional Review Board Statement: Not applicable.

Informed Consent Statement: Not applicable.

Data Availability Statement: Not applicable.

Conflicts of Interest: The authors have no relevant financial or non-financial interests to disclose.

References

1. De Haan, J.; Verheecke, M.; Van Calsteren, K.; Van Calster, B.; Shmakov, R.G.; Gziri, M.M.; Halaska, M.J.; Fruscio, R.; Lok, C.A.; Boere, I.A.; et al. Oncological management and obstetric and neonatal outcomes for women diagnosed with cancer during pregnancy: A 20-year international cohort study of 1170 patients. *Lancet Oncol.* **2018**, *19*, 337–346. [CrossRef]
2. Schirrmacher, V. From chemotherapy to biological therapy: A review of novel concepts to reduce the side effects of systemic cancer treatment. *Int. J. Oncol.* **2019**, *54*, 407–419.
3. Sohda, M.; Kuwano, H. Current status and future prospects for esophageal cancer treatment. *Ann. Thorac. Cardiovasc. Surg.* **2017**, *23*, 1–11. [CrossRef]
4. Allahyari, H.; Heidari, S.; Ghamgosha, M.; Saffarian, P.; Amani, J. Immunotoxin: A new tool for cancer therapy. *Tumor Biol.* **2017**, *39*, 1010428317692226. [CrossRef]
5. Hassan, R.; Alewine, C.; Pastan, I. New life for immunotoxin cancer therapy. *Clin. Cancer Res.* **2016**, *22*, 1055–1058. [CrossRef]
6. Dandawate, P.R.; Subramaniam, D.; Jensen, R.A.; Anant, S. (Eds.) Targeting cancer stem cells and signaling pathways by phytochemicals: Novel approach for breast cancer therapy. In *Seminars in Cancer Biology*; Elsevier: Amsterdam, The Netherlands, 2016.
7. El Hout, M.; Dos Santos, L.; Hamaï, A.; Mehrpour, M. (Eds.) A promising new approach to cancer therapy: Targeting iron metabolism in cancer stem cells. In *Seminars in Cancer Biology*; Elsevier: Amsterdam, The Netherlands, 2018.
8. Mohammadi, M.; Rezaie, E.; Sakhteman, A.; Zarei, N. A highly potential cleavable linker for tumor targeting antibody-chemokines. *J. Biomol. Struct. Dyn.* **2020**, 1–11. [CrossRef]
9. Sohrabi, E.; Moslemi, M.; Rezaie, E.; Nafissi, N.; Khaledi, M.; Afkhami, H.; Fathi, J.; Zekri, A. The tissue expression of MCT3, MCT8, and MCT9 genes in women with breast cancer. *Genes Genom.* **2021**, *43*, 1065–1077. [CrossRef]
10. Sohrabi, E.; Rezaie, E.; Heiat, M.; Sefidi-Heris, Y. An Integrated Data Analysis of mRNA, miRNA and Signaling Pathways in Pancreatic Cancer. *Biochem. Genet.* **2021**, *59*, 1326–1358. [CrossRef] [PubMed]
11. Iglesias, B.V.; Centeno, G.; Pascuccelli, H.; Ward, F.; Peters, M.G.; Puricelli, L.; Bal de Kier Joffé, E. Expression pattern of glypican-3-GPC3-during human embryonic and fetal development. *Histol. Histopathol.* **2008**, *23*, 1333–1340. [PubMed]
12. Ligato, S.; Mandich, D.; Cartun, R.W. Utility of glypican-3 in differentiating hepatocellular carcinoma from other primary and metastatic lesions in FNA of the liver: An immunocytochemical study. *Mod. Pathol.* **2008**, *21*, 626–631. [CrossRef] [PubMed]
13. Gao, W.; Kim, H.; Feng, M.; Phung, Y.; Xavier, C.P.; Rubin, J.S.; Ho, M. Inactivation of Wnt signaling by a human antibody that recognizes the heparan sulfate chains of glypican-3 for liver cancer therapy. *Hepatology* **2014**, *60*, 576–587. [CrossRef] [PubMed]
14. Gao, W.; Tang, Z.; Zhang, Y.-F.; Feng, M.; Qian, M.; Dimitrov, D.S.; Ho, M. Immunotoxin targeting glypican-3 regresses liver cancer via dual inhibition of Wnt signalling and protein synthesis. *Nat. Commun.* **2015**, *6*, 6536. [CrossRef] [PubMed]
15. Feng, M.; Gao, W.; Wang, R.; Chen, W.; Man, Y.G.; Figg, W.D.; Wang, X.W.; Dimitrov, D.S.; Ho, M. Therapeutically targeting glypican-3 via a conformation-specific single-domain antibody in hepatocellular carcinoma. *Proc. Natl. Acad. Sci. USA* **2013**, *110*, E1083–E1091. [CrossRef] [PubMed]
16. Sun, C.K.; Chua, M.-S.; He, J.; Samuel, K.S. Suppression of glypican 3 inhibits growth of hepatocellular carcinoma cells through up-regulation of TGF-β2. *Neoplasia* **2011**, *13*, 735-IN25. [CrossRef] [PubMed]
17. Mounajjed, T.; Zhang, L.; Wu, T.T. Glypican-3 expression in gastrointestinal and pancreatic epithelial neoplasms. *Hum. Pathol.* **2013**, *44*, 542–550. [CrossRef] [PubMed]
18. Moek, K.L.; Fehrmann, R.S.; van der Vegt, B.; de Vries, E.G.; de Groot, D.J. Glypican 3 overexpression across a broad spectrum of tumor types discovered with functional genomic mRNA profiling of a large cancer database. *Am. J. Pathol.* **2018**, *188*, 1973–1981. [CrossRef]

19. Keshtvarz, M.; Salimian, J.; Yaseri, M.; Bathaie, S.Z.; Rezaie, E.; Aliramezani, A.; Norouzbabaei, Z.; Amani, J.; Douraghi, M. Bioinformatic prediction and experimental validation of a PE38-based recombinant immunotoxin targeting the Fn14 receptor in cancer cells. *Immunotherapy* **2017**, *9*, 387–400. [CrossRef] [PubMed]
20. Rezaie, E.; Amani, J.; Pour, A.B.; Hosseini, H.M. A new scfv-based recombinant immunotoxin against EPHA2-overexpressing breast cancer cells; High in vitro anti-cancer potency. *Eur. J. Pharmacol.* **2020**, *870*, 172912. [CrossRef]
21. Rezaie, E.; Mohammadi, M.; Sakhteman, A.; Bemani, P.; Ahrari, S. Application of molecular dynamics simulations to design a dual-purpose oligopeptide linker sequence for fusion proteins. *J. Mol. Modeling* **2018**, *24*, 313. [CrossRef]
22. Rezaie, E.; Nekoie, H.; Miri, A.; Oulad, G.; Ahmadi, A.; Saadati, M.; Bozorgmehr, M.; Ebrahimi, M.; Salimian, J. Different frequencies of memory B-cells induced by tetanus, botulinum, and heat-labile toxin binding domains. *Microb. Pathog.* **2019**, *127*, 225–232. [CrossRef]
23. Keshtvarz, M.; Salimian, J.; Amani, J.; Douraghi, M.; Rezaie, E. In silico analysis of STX2a-PE15-P4A8 chimeric protein as a novel immunotoxin for cancer therapy. *Silico Pharmacol.* **2021**, *9*, 19. [CrossRef]
24. Rezaie, E.; Pour, A.B.; Amani, J.; Hosseini, H.M. Bioinformatics Predictions, Expression, Purification and Structural Analysis of the PE38KDEL-scfv Immunotoxin against EPHA2 Receptor. *Int. J. Pept. Res. Ther.* **2020**, *26*, 979–996. [CrossRef]
25. Bernasconi, N.L.; Traggiai, E.; Lanzavecchia, A. Maintenance of serological memory by polyclonal activation of human memory B cells. *Science* **2002**, *298*, 2199–2202. [CrossRef]
26. Fleming, B.D.; Ho, M. Glypican-3 targeting immunotoxins for the treatment of liver cancer. *Toxins* **2016**, *8*, 274. [CrossRef]
27. Wang, C.; Gao, W.; Feng, M.; Pastan, I.; Ho, M. Construction of an immunotoxin, HN3-mPE24, targeting glypican-3 for liver cancer therapy. *Oncotarget* **2017**, *8*, 32450. [CrossRef] [PubMed]
28. Zhang, Y.-F.; Ho, M. Humanization of high-affinity antibodies targeting glypican-3 in hepatocellular carcinoma. *Sci. Rep.* **2016**, *6*, 33878. [CrossRef] [PubMed]
29. Heiat, M.; Hashemi Yeganeh, H.; Alavian, S.M.; Rezaie, E. Immunotoxins Immunotherapy against Hepatocellular Carcinoma: A Promising Prospect. *Toxins* **2021**, *13*, 719. [CrossRef]
30. Ogawa, K.; Tanaka, S.; Matsumura, S.; Murakata, A.; Ban, D.; Ochiai, T.; Irie, T.; Kudo, A.; Nakamura, N.; Tanabe, M.; et al. EpCAM-Targeted Therapy for Human Hepatocellular Carcinoma. *Ann. Surg. Oncol.* **2014**, *21*, 1314–1322. [CrossRef]
31. Liu, Z.; Feng, Z.; Zhu, X.; Xu, W.; Zhu, J.; Zhang, X.; Fan, Z.; Ji, G. Construction, expression, and characterization of an anti-tumor immunotoxin containing the human anti-c-Met single-chain antibody and PE38KDEL. *Immunol. Lett.* **2013**, *149*, 30–40. [CrossRef]
32. Lv, M.; Qiu, F.; Li, T.; Sun, Y.; Zhang, C.; Zhu, P.; Qi, X.; Wan, J.; Yang, K.; Zhang, K. Construction, expression, and characterization of a recombinant immunotoxin targeting EpCAM. *Mediat. Inflamm.* **2015**, *2015*, 460264. [CrossRef]
33. Marvig, R.L.; Sommer, L.M.M.; Molin, S.; Johansen, H.K. Convergent evolution and adaptation of Pseudomonas aeruginosa within patients with cystic fibrosis. *Nat. Genet.* **2015**, *47*, 57–64. [CrossRef]
34. Michalska, M.; Wolf, P. Pseudomonas Exotoxin A: Optimized by evolution for effective killing. *Front. Microbiol.* **2015**, *6*, 963. [CrossRef]
35. Majtnerová, P.; Roušar, T. An overview of apoptosis assays detecting DNA fragmentation. *Mol. Biol. Rep.* **2018**, *45*, 1469–1478. [CrossRef]
36. Decker, T.; Oelsner, M.; Kreitman, R.J.; Salvatore, G.; Wang, Q.-C.; Pastan, I.; Peschel, C.; Licht, T. Induction of caspase-dependent programmed cell death in B-cell chronic lymphocytic leukemia by anti-CD22 immunotoxins. *Blood* **2004**, *103*, 2718–2726. [CrossRef]
37. Keppler-Hafkemeyer, A.; Brinkmann, U.; Pastan, I. Role of caspases in immunotoxin-induced apoptosis of cancer cells. *Biochemistry* **1998**, *37*, 16934–16942. [CrossRef]
38. Mathew, M.; Zaineb, K.; Verma, R.S. GM-CSF-DFF40: A novel humanized immunotoxin induces apoptosis in acute myeloid leukemia cells. *Apoptosis* **2013**, *18*, 882–895. [CrossRef] [PubMed]
39. Yang, Y.; Tian, Z.; Ding, Y.; Li, X.; Zhang, Z.; Yang, L.; Zhao, F.; Ren, F.; Guo, R. EGFR-targeted immunotoxin exerts antitumor effects on esophageal cancers by increasing ROS accumulation and inducing apoptosis via inhibition of the Nrf2-Keap1 pathway. *J. Immunol. Res.* **2018**, *2018*, 1090287. [CrossRef]
40. Simon, H.-U.; Haj-Yehia, A.; Levi-Schaffer, F. Role of reactive oxygen species (ROS) in apoptosis induction. *Apoptosis* **2000**, *5*, 415–418. [CrossRef] [PubMed]
41. Zhou, L.-J.; Zhu, X.-Z. Reactive oxygen species-induced apoptosis in PC12 cells and protective effect of bilobalide. *J. Pharmacol. Exp. Ther.* **2000**, *293*, 982–988. [PubMed]
42. Ghetie, M.-A.; Picker, L.J.; Richardson, J.A.; Tucker, K.; Uhr, J.W.; Vitetta, E.S. Anti-CD19 inhibits the growth of human B-cell tumor lines in vitro and of Daudi cells in SCID mice by inducing cell cycle arrest. *Blood* **1994**, *83*, 1329–1336. [CrossRef]
43. Mohamed, M.F.; Wood, S.J.; Roy, R.; Reiser, J.; Kuzel, T.M.; Shafikhani, S.H. Pseudomonas aeruginosa ExoT induces G1 cell cycle arrest in melanoma cells. *Cell. Microbiol.* **2021**, *23*, e13339. [CrossRef] [PubMed]
44. Zhang, C.; Cai, Y.; Dai, X.; Wu, J.; Lan, Y.; Zhang, H.; Lu, M.; Liu, J.; Xie, J. Novel EGFR-bispecific recombinant immunotoxin based on cucurmosin shows potent anti-tumor efficiency in vitro. *Oncol. Rep.* **2021**, *45*, 493–500. [CrossRef] [PubMed]
45. Basu, A.; Haldar, S. The relationship between BcI2, Bax and p53: Consequences for cell cycle progression and cell death. *Mol. Hum. Reprod.* **1998**, *4*, 1099–1109. [CrossRef] [PubMed]

46. Yuan, X.; Zhou, Y.; Casanova, E.; Chai, M.; Kiss, E.; Gröne, H.-J.; Schütz, G.; Grummt, I. Genetic inactivation of the transcription factor TIF-IA leads to nucleolar disruption, cell cycle arrest, and p53-mediated apoptosis. *Mol. Cell* **2005**, *19*, 77–87. [CrossRef] [PubMed]
47. Bacac, M.; Stamenkovic, I. Metastatic cancer cell. *Annu. Rev. Pathol.* **2008**, *3*, 221–247. [CrossRef] [PubMed]
48. Bruell, D.; Stöcker, M.; Huhn, M.; Redding, N.; Küpper, M.; Schumacher, P.; Paetz, A.; Bruns, C.J.; Haisma, H.J.; Fischer, R.; et al. The recombinant anti-EGF receptor immunotoxin 425(scFv)-ETA′ suppresses growth of a highly metastatic pancreatic carcinoma cell line. *Int. J. Oncol.* **2003**, *23*, 1179–1186. [CrossRef] [PubMed]
49. Bayat, S.; Zeinoddini, M.; Azizi, A.; Khalili, M.A.N. Co-solvents effects on the stability of recombinant immunotoxin denileukin diftitox: Structure and function assessment. *Iran. J. Sci. Technol. Trans. A Sci.* **2019**, *43*, 2091–2097. [CrossRef]

toxins

MDPI

Article

Sequence, Structure, and Binding Site Analysis of Kirkiin in Comparison with Ricin and Other Type 2 RIPs

Stefania Maiello [1,†], Rosario Iglesias [2,*,†], Letizia Polito [1,*], Lucía Citores [2], Massimo Bortolotti [1], José M. Ferreras [2,‡] and Andrea Bolognesi [1,‡]

1 Department of Experimental, Diagnostic and Specialty Medicine—DIMES, Alma Mater Studiorum—University of Bologna, Via S. Giacomo 14, 40126 Bologna, Italy; stefania.maiello2@unibo.it (S.M.); massimo.bortolotti2@unibo.it (M.B.); andrea.bolognesi@unibo.it (A.B.)

2 Department of Biochemistry and Molecular Biology and Physiology, Faculty of Sciences, University of Valladolid, 47011 Valladolid, Spain; lucia.citores@uva.es (L.C.); josemiguel.ferreras@uva.es (J.M.F.)

* Correspondence: riglesia@bio.uva.es (R.I.); letizia.polito@unibo.it (L.P.)

† These authors contributed equally to this work.

‡ Co-senior authorship.

Abstract: Kirkiin is a new type 2 ribosome-inactivating protein (RIP) purified from the caudex of *Adenia kirkii* with a cytotoxicity compared to that of stenodactylin. The high toxicity of RIPs from *Adenia* genus plants makes them interesting tools for biotechnology and therapeutic applications, particularly in cancer therapy. The complete amino acid sequence and 3D structure prediction of kirkiin are here reported. Gene sequence analysis revealed that kirkiin is encoded by a 1572 bp open reading frame, corresponding to 524 amino acid residues, without introns. The amino acid sequence analysis showed a high degree of identity with other *Adenia* RIPs. The 3D structure of kirkiin preserves the overall folding of type 2 RIPs. The key amino acids of the active site, described for ricin and other RIPs, are also conserved in the kirkiin A chain. Sugar affinity studies and docking experiments revealed that both the 1α and 2γ sites of the kirkiin B chain exhibit binding activity toward lactose and D-galactose, being lower than ricin. The replacement of His246 in the kirkiin 2γ site instead of Tyr248 in ricin causes a different structure arrangement that could explain the lower sugar affinity of kirkiin with respect to ricin.

Keywords: 3D structure; plant toxin; primary sequence; ribosome-inactivating protein; kirkiin; ricin; toxic lectin; sugar specificity; cancer therapy

Key Contribution: The knowledge of amino acid sequence and the 3D structure prediction of kirkiin are essential because of its potential in medicine, for cancer treatment, and of its biotechnological applications in neuroscience. Moreover, the comparison between the structural properties of kirkiin and those of other type 2 RIPs could be useful for explaining the differences in enzymatic activity and toxicity.

Citation: Maiello, S.; Iglesias, R.; Polito, L.; Citores, L.; Bortolotti, M.; Ferreras, J.M.; Bolognesi, A. Sequence, Structure, and Binding Site Analysis of Kirkiin in Comparison with Ricin and Other Type 2 RIPs. *Toxins* **2021**, *13*, 862. https://doi.org/10.3390/toxins13120862

Received: 22 October 2021
Accepted: 30 November 2021
Published: 3 December 2021

1. Introduction

Ribosome-inactivating proteins (RIPs) are plant toxic enzymes widely distributed in nature, and many RIP-containing plants have been used for centuries in traditional and folk medicine for the treatment of several pathologies [1,2]. Type 2 RIPs consist of two polypeptide chains, called A and B chain, which are linked together through a disulfide bridge. The A chain possesses rRNA N-glycosylase and polynucleotide:adenosine glycosidase activities that irreversibly damage rRNA and other polynucleotide substrates inside the cells, thus causing cell death [3]. The B chain has lectin properties, which allows type 2 RIPs to bind the galactoside residues on cell membrane, facilitating the entry into cells and resulting in high cytotoxicity.

Type 2 RIPs extracted from *Adenia* genus plants are the most potent plant toxins known to date, being able to irreversibly inhibit protein synthesis and to induce cell death at very low concentrations. In addition, *Adenia* RIPs proved very toxic for animals at small doses. This high toxicity is due to the peculiarity of *Adenia* toxins to be transported in a retrograde manner both along peripheral nerves, in the same way as ricin and abrin, and within the central nervous system [4,5]. This property could have different medical and biotechnological applications in the field of neuroscience to selectively lesion specific neurons, i.e., in behavior studies. The most toxic *Adenia* RIP is stenodactylin, which induces several molecular mechanisms triggering different cell death pathways [6,7]. Recently, kirkiin, a new type 2 RIP from the caudex of *Adenia kirkii*, was purified and characterized, showing a cytotoxicity comparable to that of stenodactylin. Kirkiin has N-glycosylase activity against mammalian and yeast ribosomes, and it is able to completely inhibit protein synthesis both in a cell-free system and in cells, and to induce cell death by apoptosis at very low doses in the human neuroblastoma cell line [8]. Due to its elevated cytotoxicity, it can be considered an attractive molecule for the production of immunotoxins for the treatment of cancers, and as a single agent for loco-regional treatments [7,9,10].

This study investigates the primary sequence of kirkiin, and a comparison with the sequences of other type 2 RIPs from *Adenia* species and ricin was performed, in order to provide useful information about the amino acids directly or indirectly involved in kirkiin toxicity. A three-dimensional structure was also predicted through homology modeling. Knowledge about the amino acid sequence associated with the structure analysis is essential to understand the protein function and to investigate structure–function relationships in the mechanism of action of kirkiin. Moreover, the carbohydrate-binding properties of kirkiin were here investigated in order to better understand the correlation between structure and function of the molecule.

2. Results

2.1. Isolation and Cloning of Kirkiin Gene

The kirkiin gene sequence was determined by PCR amplification of *A. kirkii* genomic DNA. Based on the N- and C-terminal amino acid sequences of other RIPs derived from plants of *Adenia* genus (modeccin, lanceolin 1, lanceolin 2, stenodactylin, and volkensin) and on the information available in GenBank on volkensin amino acid sequence (CAD61022) and stenodactylin (MT580807), four specific primers were designed for PCR amplification of the kirkiin gene (see Section 4.2.2). Two primer pairs amplified two genomic DNA fragments corresponding to the A chain (A2-B1R) and the entire sequence of kirkiin (A2-B5R). The information obtained on the sequence was analyzed using the algorithms available on http://expasy.org (accessed on 15 October 2021) [11]. Excluding the nucleotide sequence coding for the signal peptide, the DNA sequence analysis revealed that kirkiin is encoded by a 1572 bp open reading frame (ORF) without introns, encoding a protein of 524 amino acids (Figure 1). The N-terminal sequence of kirkiin A chain was determined by direct Edman degradation and allowed us to obtain the sequence of the first 15 amino acid residues for the A chain (see below). As a control, also, the N-terminal sequence of the B chain was determined to confirm the method validity; the sequence deduced from the chemical sequencing perfectly matched the nucleotide sequence. The gene contains the 753 bp sequence encoding the A chain (251 amino acids with a theoretical molecular weight (Mw) of 28,324.21) and 774 bp sequence encoding the B chain (258 amino acids with a theoretical Mw of 28,506.13), which were separated by a sequence linker of 45 bp. The C-terminal end of the A chain and the linker sequence were estimated on the basis of the homology with other toxic type 2 RIPs from the same genus.

```
nnnnnnnnnnnnnnnnnnnnnnnnnnnnnnnnngccacggtagagaggtacactcagttt   60
 V  F  P  K  V  I  L  D  C  T  R  A  T  V  E  R  Y  T  Q  F    20
ataatgctcttaaggaacgaactggcgggtgatgtttctccacagggaatacgcaggctg  120
 I  M  L  L  R  N  E  L  A  G  D  V  S  P  Q  G  I  R  R  L    40
aggaatccggctgatattcagccttcacagcgttttattcttatacaactcaacggcttc  180
 R  N  P  A  D  I  Q  P  S  Q  R  F  I  L  I  Q  L  N  G  F    60
gtaggctccgtcaccttgataatggacgtcagcaatgcgtatctattgggttatgagagc  240
 V  G  S  V  T  L  I  M  D  V  S  N  A  Y  L  L  G  Y  E  S    80
cgcaactttgtgtatcacttcaacgatgtctctacctcttcgatcgccgatgttttccca  300
 R  N  F  V  Y  H  F  N  D  V  S  T  S  S  I  A  D  V  F  P   100
gacgtacaacgtcaacagttgccatttgaaggcggctatcccagcatgcgacactatgcg  360
 D  V  Q  R  Q  Q  L  P  F  E  G  G  Y  P  S  M  R  H  Y  A   120
ccggagagagatcaaattgaccacggattcatcgaactggcatacgctgttgatacgctc  420
 P  E  R  D  Q  I  D  H  G  F  I  E  L  A  Y  A  V  D  T  L   140
tactatagtagtcaaggctacgaacagatcgcgcgttcactcgtgctctgcgccgggatg  480
 Y  Y  S  S  Q  G  Y  E  Q  I  A  R  S  L  V  L  C  A  G  M   160
gttgcagaagccgcccggttccgctacatcgagggcctggtgcgtcaaagcattgtcggg  540
 V  A  E  A  A  R  F  R  Y  I  E  G  L  V  R  Q  S  I  V  G   180
ccaggagactacggaactttcagaccggatgcgttgatgtactcagtcgtgacagcgtgg  600
 P  G  D  Y  G  T  F  R  P  D  A  L  M  Y  S  V  V  T  A  W   200
cagactctttcagaaagaatccagggatccttcgacggagctttccagccagttcagctg  660
 Q  T  L  S  E  R  I  Q  G  S  F  D  G  A  F  Q  P  V  Q  L   220
gggtatgccagcgatccctttattgggacaacgtcgcacaggccatcaccaggctgtca  720
 G  Y  A  S  D  P  F  Y  W  D  N  V  A  Q  A  I  T  R  L  S   240
ctcatgctattcgcctgcgctaaacctccaaggcaatccgattcccccatggtgataagg  780
 L  M  L  F  A  C  A  K  P  P  R  Q  S  D  S  P  M  V  I  R   251
tcctttgtggataggaacgatcctgtctgcccttccggggagacgactgcgtacatcgtg  840
 S  F  V  D  R  N  D  P  V  C  P  S  G  E  T  T  A  Y  I  V    14
gggcgggacgggcgctgtgtggacgtgaaggatgaggaattcttcgacggcaataaagta  900
 G  R  D  G  R  C  V  D  V  K  D  E  E  F  F  D  G  N  K  V    34
cagatgtggccgtgcaagtccagccagaatgcaaaccagctgtggactataaagagagac  960
 Q  M  W  P  C  K  S  S  Q  N  A  N  Q  L  W  T  I  K  R  D    54
ggcactattcggtgcaagggaaagtgcttgactgtgaggagcccgcaactgtacgctatg 1020
 G  T  I  R  C  K  G  K  C  L  T  V  R  S  P  Q  L  Y  A  M    74
atctggaactgcaccacttttatgctcctgccaccaagtgggaagtgtgggacaacggg 1080
 I  W  N  C  T  T  F  Y  A  P  A  T  K  W  E  V  W  D  N  G    94
accatcatcaaccccgcctccgggagggtgttgaccgcgtccactggggacgcgggcgtc 1140
 T  I  I  N  P  A  S  G  R  V  L  T  A  S  T  G  D  A  G  V   114
gtcctcagcctggagcacaacgagaacgccgctagccaggcgtggagagtgaccaatgtg 1200
 V  L  S  L  E  H  N  E  N  A  A  S  Q  A  W  R  V  T  N  V   134
acagcacctacggtgacaaccattgtgggatatgatgatctctgcctggaaaccaacgac 1260
 T  A  P  T  V  T  T  I  V  G  Y  D  D  L  C  L  E  T  N  D   154
agcaatgtatggttggccaactgcgtgaaaggcaagacgcaacagagatgggcgcagtat 1320
 S  N  V  W  L  A  N  C  V  K  G  K  T  Q  Q  R  W  A  Q  Y   174
gcggatggcaccatacgctcccagtccagcctcagcaaatgcctcacctgcagtggcgac 1380
 A  D  G  T  I  R  S  Q  S  S  L  S  K  C  L  T  C  S  G  D   194
tgcgtcaagctggcaaagatcgtcaacacggactgtgctggatccgccttgagccgttgg 1440
 C  V  K  L  A  K  I  V  N  T  D  C  A  G  S  A  L  S  R  W   214
tacttcaacacctttggcggcatcgtgaatctgttgaccgacatggtgatggacgtgaaa 1500
 Y  F  N  T  F  G  G  I  V  N  L  L  T  D  M  V  M  D  V  K   234
gagtccaatccgagtctcaacgaaataattgcccacccgtggcatggaaactccaaccag 1560
 E  S  N  P  S  L  N  E  I  I  A  H  P  W  H  G  N  S  N  Q   254
caatggttccta 1572
 Q  W  F  L   258
```

Figure 1. Full-length sequence and derived amino acid sequence of the kirkiin gene. The A chain is represented in black, the B chain is represented in blue, and the sequence of the linker peptide is represented in red. The N-terminal amino acid sequences of the A and B chains obtained by Edman degradation are underlined. Numbering refers to the position of the amino acids in the mature A and B chains. The DNA sequence for kirkiin was submitted to GenBank (accession number: OK283399). The letter "n" means "unknown nucleotide residue", being the amino acid sequence obtained exclusively by Edman degradation.

The protein sequence alignment between the N-terminal sequences obtained for kirkiin and those already known for modeccin [12] (*A. digitata*), volkensin [13] (*A. volkensii*), lanceolin 1, lanceolin 2 (*A. lanceolata*), and stenodactylin (*A. stenodactyla*) [14] showed that kirkiin A chain shares 14/15 amino acids with stenodactylin and lanceolin A2. The different amino acid residue is Phe at position 7 in stenodactylin A chain, which is replaced by Leu in kirkiin A chain. This substitution is also present in the A chains of modeccin and in lanceolin 1. Moreover, all the N-terminal amino acid sequences of *Adenia* RIPs, except for volkensin, present a Cys residue at position 9 (position 8 for lanceolin A1). The identity among the B chains is very high, except for the first three N-terminal residues Asp-Pro-Val that are present in kirkiin as well as in volkensin and stenodactylin B chains but not in modeccin and lanceolin (Figure 2).

```
Modeccin A chain        -FPKVTLDDTRATVESYTT--- 18
Lanceolin A1            -FPKVILDCTRATVERYTQFI- 20
Lanceolin A2            VFPKVIFDCTRATVERYTQFI- 21
Volkensin A chain       VFPKVPFDVPKATVESYTRFIR 22
Stenodactylin A chain   VFPKVIFDCTRATVERYTQFIM 22
Kirkiin A chain         VFPKVILDCTRATVE------- 15
                         **** :*  :****


Modeccin B chain        EMICPSGETTAYIVGRXGXXV  21
Lanceolin B1            --DCPFGETTAYIVGRDXXCV  19
Lanceolin B2            --DCPSGETTAYIVGRDXXCV  19
Volkensin B chain       DPVCPSGETTAFIVGRDGRCV  21
Stenodactylin B chain   DPVCPSGETTAYIVGRDXXXV  21
Kirkiin B chain         DPVCPSGETT-----------  10
                           ** ****
```

Figure 2. Amino acid alignment of the N-terminal sequences of modeccin, lanceolin, stenodactylin, volkensin, and kirkiin. Identical residues (*), conserved substitutions (:) are reported. X, unassigned amino acid positions [15].

A multiple sequence alignment was performed between *Adenia* RIPs (kirkiin, stenodactylin, and volkensin) and ricin, which is the best-known RIP [16], using the program Clustal Omega [15] (Figure 3). The amino acid comparison showed a higher identity of kirkiin with RIPs purified from plants belonging to the same genus (96.3% with stenodactylin and 87% with volkensin) with respect to ricin (40.4%). The alignment between kirkiin and stenodactylin showed a higher identity of A chains (97.6%) in comparison to B chains (95.4%). On the contrary, the alignment between the kirkiin sequence and those of volkensin and ricin showed a higher identity of the B chains (89.2% with volkensin and 48.4% with ricin) with respect to the A chains (84.4% with volkensin and 35.1% with ricin). Similarly to stenodactylin, kirkiin contains a total of 15 cysteinyl residues, which is one more than that present in volkensin and four more than ricin. The kirkiin A chain includes three cysteinyl residues at the positions 9, 157, and 246. The B chain includes 12 cysteinyl residues (at positions 4, 20, 39, 59, 63, 78, 149, 162, 188, 191, 195, and 206). It is known for other type 2 RIPs, such as ricin [17], that the N-terminal cysteine of the B chain (Cys4) forms an interchain disulfide bridge with the cysteine at the C-terminal of the A chain (Cys246), and that eight cysteines in the B chain (Cys20-Cys39, Cys63-Cys78, Cys149-Cys162, and Cys188-Cys206) form conserved intramolecular disulfide bridges. Two possible glycosylation sites in the kirkiin B chain were identified by the program NetNGlyc1.0 [18] at position Asn93-Gly94-Thr95 and Asn133-Val134-Thr135. The amino acid residues reported to be involved in the active site of RIPs are conserved within the sequence of kirkiin and stenodactylin A chains, except for Ala199 and Ala245, which are replaced with Gln198 and Val244 in volkensin. All the amino acids present in sugar binding sites are conserved in the kirkiin B chain, similarly to stenodactylin and volkensin (Figure 3).

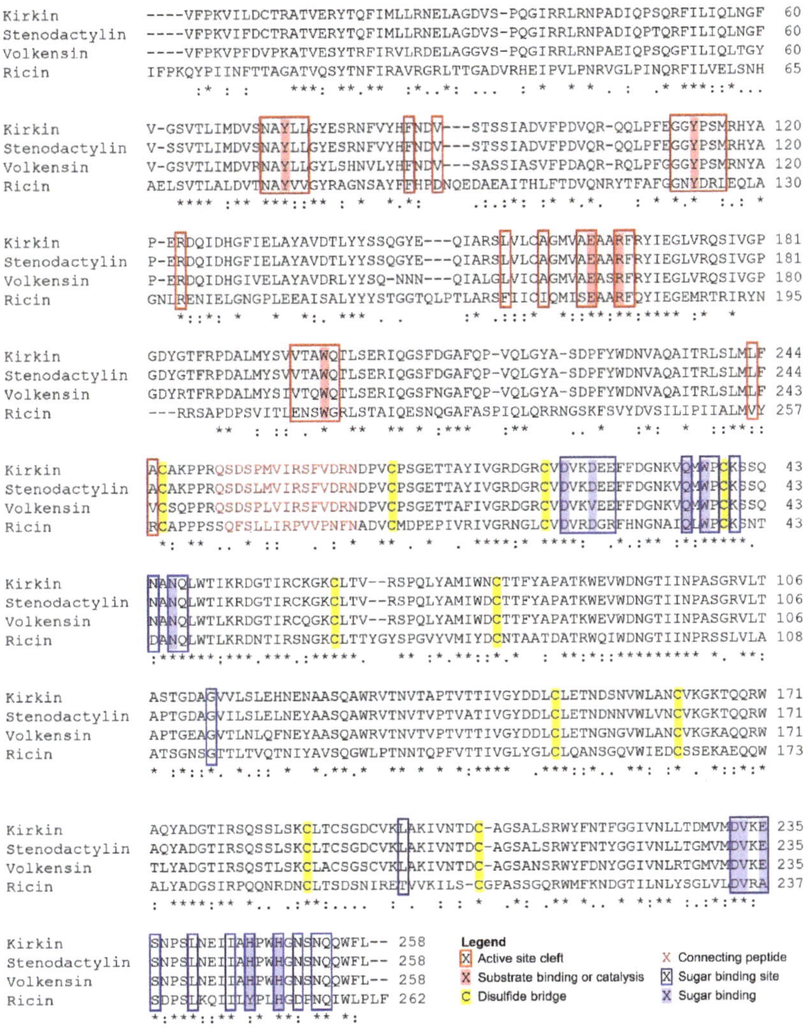

Figure 3. Alignment between kirkiin, stenodactylin (GenBank MT580807), volkensin (GenBank CAD61022), and ricin (GenBank P02879). Identical residues (*), conserved substitutions (:), and semiconserved substitutions (.) are reported. The A and B chains are written in black letters; the sequence of the linker peptide is in red. The putative amino acids that are present in the active site pocket (boxed in red) or in the galactoside-binding sites (boxed in blue), those involved in substrate binding or catalysis (highlighted in red), those involved in sugar binding (highlighted in blue), and those involved in disulfide bridges (highlighted in yellow) are represented, and they were assigned by comparison with the structure of ricin (PDB accession no. 2AAI, 3RTI, and 3RTJ). The dash indicates a gap introduced into the sequences to maximize alignments.

2.2. Structural Analysis of Kirkiin

Given the availability of the complete amino acid sequence, it was possible to predict the three-dimensional structure of kirkiin with a computational model using several type 2 RIP crystal structures as templates. The best three-dimensional model obtained for kirkiin is shown in Figure 4a, and it was found to have a confidence score (C-score) of 0.61, template modelling (Tm) score of 0.80 ± 0.09, and root-mean-square deviation (RMSD) of

6.1 ± 3.8 Å, which satisfied the range of parameters for molecular modeling. The overall folding of type 2 RIPs is conserved in kirkiin, apart from a few discrepancies due to some deletions and insertions in loop regions. The kirkiin A chain structure consists of three folding domains. The first domain includes the N-terminus until the residue Phe109, with the first four residues not structured. It is composed of six antiparallel β-sheets (strands from a to f) and two α-helices (helices A and B) alternating in the order aAbcdeBf (Figure 4b). Tyr74, one of the amino acids directly involved in the binding of adenine, is located in the first domain. The second domain extends from Glu110 to Ala199 and consists of five α-helices (helices from C to G), with a classical helix–loop–helix motif. The second amino acid involved in adenine binding (Tyr113) and the catalytic amino acids (Glu163 and Arg166) are located here. The last domain consists of two α-helices and two antiparallel β-sheets in a α-helix–β-fork–α-helix motif (HghI), ending with an unstructured coil region in the C-terminus. This structural motif seems to be important for the interaction of RIPs with cell membranes [19] and for the explanation of their biological and toxic activities [20], and it contains the residue Trp200 of the active site. The three folding domains of the A chain form a deep pocket which accommodates the conserved active site. Similar to other type 2 RIPs, the kirkiin B chain is made of two homologous globular lectin domains arisen by gene duplication [21], which is exclusively formed by β-sheets. Each domain consists of four homologous subdomains (1λ, 1α, 1β, and 1γ for lectin 1; 2λ, 2α, 2β, and 2γ for lectin 2). The subdomains 1λ (from the B chain N-terminus to residue Thr9) and 2λ (residues Val131 to Pro137) are responsible for the binding to the A chain and for the interconnection between the two B chain domains, respectively. The subdomains 1α (residues Thr10 to Thr56), 1β (residues Ile57 to Gly94), and 1γ (residues Thr95 to Asn130) are arranged in a trefoil structure. This arrangement is also present in lectin 2 with subdomains 2α (residues Thr138 to Thr178), 2β (residues Ile179 to Gly221), and 2γ (Ile222 to Leu258) (Figure 4b). The subdomains 1α and 2γ contain the two galactose binding sites.

2.3. Carbohydrate Binding Properties of Kirkiin

Kirkiin showed hemagglutination activity (HA) on human A, B, and 0 erythrocytes being the minimum concentration required for activity of 0.175 mg/mL for both the A and 0 blood groups, and of 0.35 mg/mL for the B blood group (data not shown). To understand the sugar binding specificity of kirkiin, the inhibition of hemagglutination was carried out with several monosaccharides and disaccharides (Table 1). The results showed that the HA of kirkiin was inhibited by D-galactose and its derivative lactose at very similar concentrations (0.012 and 0.011 M, respectively). No affinity for D-glucose, D-fructose, D-mannose, D-sorbitol, D-mannitol, L-fucose, N-Acetyl-D-mannosamine, and sucrose was observed by kirkiin at the maximum sugar concentration tested. D-galactose was able to inhibit kirkiin HA at concentration one titer lower than that of stenodactylin (0.023 M), while lactose has the same inhibiting power for both *Adenia* RIPs. Lactose was a better inhibitor than D-galactose of stenodactylin HA, which is in agreement with previous results [14]. Lactose and D-galactose were also the best inhibitors of ricin HA; in this case, the HA inhibition was observable at very low concentrations, 2–3 titers (D-galactose) and 5 titers (lactose) lower than those of kirkiin and stenodactylin, respectively. Very low affinity was observed with D-glucose, D-fructose, D-mannose, D-sorbitol, and L-fucose in agreement with previous results [23].

a

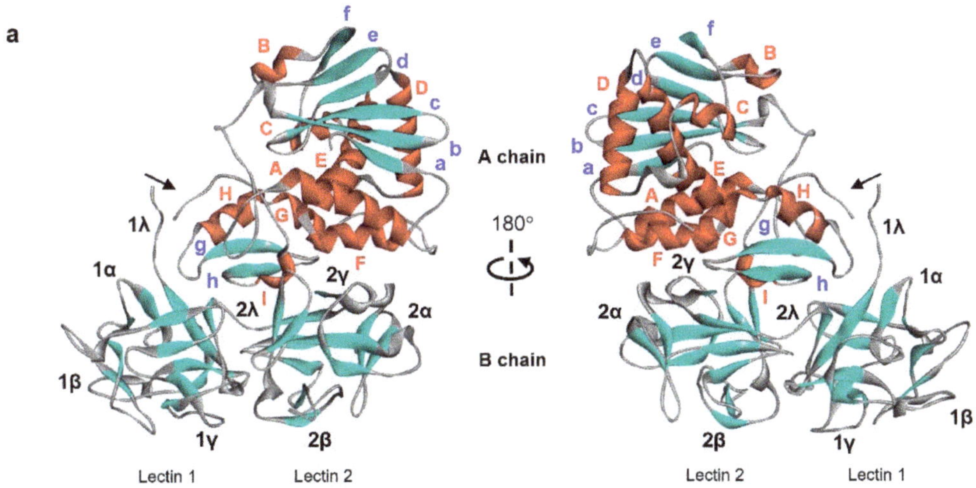

b

A chain

```
                  a         A                                                   b          c           d          e
Kirkiin      ----VFPKVILDCTRATVERYTQFIMLLRNELAGDV-SPQGIRRLRNPADIQPSQRFILIQLNGFV-GSVTLIMDVSNAYLLGYESRNFV  84
Stenodactylin ----VFPKVIFDCTRATVERYTQFIMLLRNELAGDV-SPQGIRRLRNPADIQPTQRFILIQLNGFV-SSVTLIMDVSNAYLLGYESRNFV  84
Ricin        IFPKQYPIINFTTAGATVQSYTNFIRAVRGRLTTGADVRHEIPVLPNRVGLPINQRFILVELSNHAEL SVTLALDVTNAYVVGYRAGNSA  90
                 :* : :  : ***: **:**  :*..*: ..   : *  * * ..:  .*****::*....  **** :**:***::**.: * .

                         B        f         C                    D                    E
Kirkiin      YHFNDVS---TSSIADVFPDVQR-QQLPFEGGYPSMRHYAP-ERDQIDHGFIELAYAVDTLYYSSQGY---EQIARSLVLCAGMVAEAAR 166
Stenodactylin YHFNDVS---TSSIADVFPDVQR-QQLPFEGGYPSMRHYAP-ERDQIDHGFIELAYAVDTLYYSSQGY---EQIARSLVLCAGMVAEAAR 166
Ricin        YFFHPDNQEDAEAITHLFTDVQNRYTFAFGGNYDRLEQLAGNLRENIELGNGPLEEAISALYYYSTGGTQLPTLARSFIICIQMISEAAR 180
             *.*:  .   :.:*:.:* ***.   : * *.*  :.: *   *::*: *   *  *:.:*** * *      :***:::*  *::****

             F                 G       H                g           h       I
Kirkiin      FRYIEGLVRQSIVGPGDYGTFRPDALMYSVVTAWQTLSERIQGSFDGAFQ-PVQLGYA-SDPFYWDNVAQAITRLSLMLFACAKPPR--- 251
Stenodactylin FRYIEGLVRQSIVGPGDYGTFRPDALMYSVVTAWQTLSERIQGSFDGAFQ-PVQLGYA-SDPFYWDNVAQAITRLSLMLFACAKPPR--- 251
Ricin        FQYIEGEMRTRIRYNR---RSAPDPSVITLENSWGRLSTAIQESNQGAFASPIQLQRRNGSKFSVYDVSILIPIIALMVYRCAPPPSSQF 267
             *:**** :*  *               **  : :: .:*  **  ** * :***  *:**     .. *   :*:  *  ::**:: ** **
```

B chain

```
              1λ       1α                               1β
Kirkiin       DPVCPSGETTAYIVGRDGRCVDVKDEEFFDGNKVQMWPCKSSQNANQLWTIKRDGTIRCKGKCLTV--RSPQLYAMIWNCTTFYAPAT  85
Stenodactylin DPVCPSGETTAYIVGRDGRCVDVKDEEFFDGNKVQMWPCKSSQNANQLWTIKRDGTIRCKGKCLTV--RSPQLYAMIWDCTTFYAPAT  85
Ricin         ADVCMDPEPIVRIVGRNGLCVDVRDGRFHNGNAIQLWPCKSNTDANQLWTLKRDNTIRSNGKCLTTYGYSPGVYVMIYDCNTAATDAT  87
                ** . *  . ****:* ****:* .*.:** :*:*****. :******:***.***.:*****.   ** :*.**::*.*  : **

                      1γ                                2λ  2α
Kirkiin       TKWEVWDNGTIINPASGRVLTASTGDAGVVLSLEHNENAASQAWRVTNVTAPTVTTIVGYDDLCLETNDSNVWLANCVKGKTQQRWAQ 173
Stenodactylin TKWEVWDNGTIINPASGRVLTAPTGDAGVILSLELNEYAASQAWRVTNVTVPTVATIVGYDDLCLETNDNNVWLVNCVKGKTQQRWAQ 173
Ricin         TRWQIWDNGTIINPRSSLVLAATSGNSGTTLTVQTNIYAVSQGWLPTNNTQPFVTTIVGLYGLCLQANSGQVWIEDCSSEKAEQQWAL 175
              *:*::********** *. **:* :*::*. *::: *  *.**.*  ** * * *:****  .***::*..:**: :* . *::*:**

                   2β                                 2γ
Kirkiin       YADGTIRSQSSLSKCLTCSGDCVKLAKIVNTDC-AGSALSRWYFNTFGGIVNLLTDMVMDVKESNPSLNEIIAHPWHGNSNQQWFL-- 258
Stenodactylin YADGTIRSQSSLSKCLTCSGDCVKLAKIVNTDC-AGSALSRWYFNTYGGIVNLLTGMVMDVKESNPSLNEIIAHPWHGNSNQQWFL-- 258
Ricin         YADGSIRPQQNRDNCLTSDSNIRETVVKILS-CGPASSGQRWMFKNDGTILNLYSGLVLDVRASDPSLKQIILYPLHGDPNQIWLPLF 262
               ****:** *.. .:***...:  : .  :  *  .*: .** *:. * *:** :.:*:**: *:***::** :* **: ** *:
```

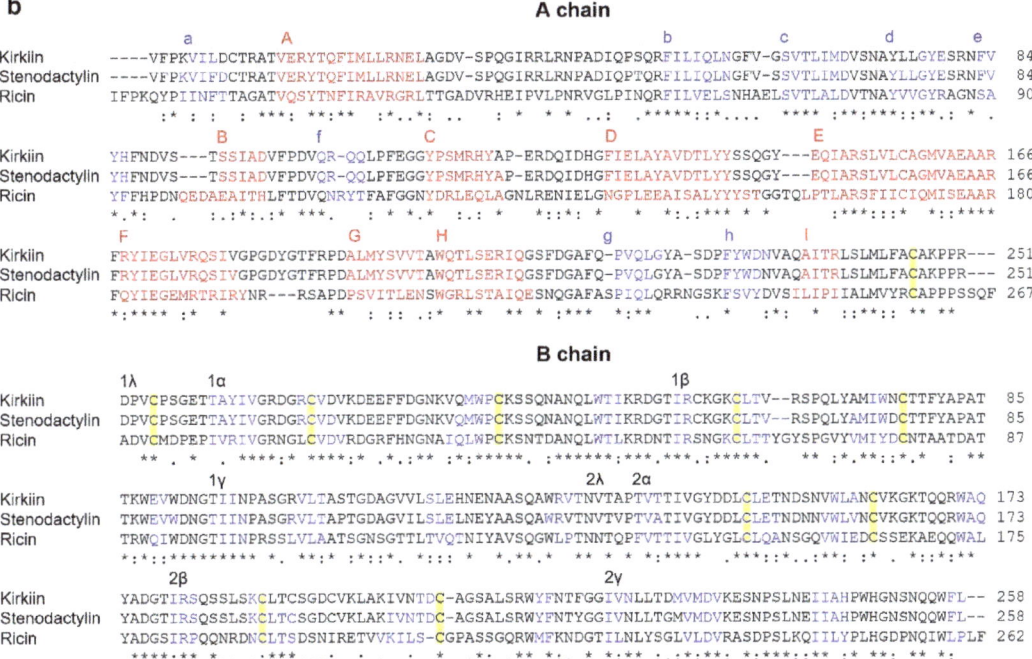

Figure 4. Structure of kirkiin. (**a**) Three-dimensional structure of kirkiin. The three-dimensional structural modeling was carried out on the I-TASSER server, and the figure was generated using Discovery Studio 2016. The α helices (red), the β chains (cyan), and the coils (gray) are represented. Arrows indicate the position of the disulfide bond linking A and B chains. (**b**) Amino acid sequence alignment of the A and B chains of kirkiin, stenodactylin, and ricin [22]. The strands (blue), the helices (red), and the cysteines involved in the disulfide bonds (highlighted in yellow) are indicated. The helices are labeled from A to I, and the strands of the β sheets are labeled from a to h in the A chain. The structural subdomains in the B chain are also indicated. Identical residues (*), conserved substitutions (:), and semiconserved substitutions (.) are reported.

Table 1. Inhibition of the hemagglutination activity of kirkiin, stenodactylin, and ricin by sugars.

Carbohydrates	Minimum Concentration Inhibiting Hemagglutination (M)		
	Kirkiin	Stenodactylin	Ricin
D-glucose	NI	1.6	1.6
D-galactose	0.012	0.023	0.0029
D-fructose	NI	NI	1.6
D-mannose	NI	NI	1.5
D-sorbitol	NI	NI	1.45
D-mannitol	NI	NI	NI
L-fucose	NI	NI	0.28
N-Acetyl-D-mannosamine	NI	NI	NI
Lactose	0.011	0.011	0.00068
Sucrose	NI	NI	NI

NI = no inhibition of hemagglutination at the maximum sugar concentration tested.

2.4. Molecular Docking

As shown in Figure 3, the sequences of the sugar binding sites of kirkiin are similar to those of stenodactylin and volkensin. The amino acids in the pockets of 1α and 2γ sites are identical in all three proteins with the exception of Asp25 of kirkiin and stenodactylin, which is Val25 in volkensin. This agrees with the finding that kirkiin and stenodactylin have similar affinities for D-galactose and lactose (Table 1). However, there are differences with ricin sugar-binding sites. So, at the 1α site, there are 10 identical amino acids out of the 14 that compose the binding pocket [22], that is 71.4%, while in the 2γ site, there are eight identical amino acids out of the 13 that make up the binding pocket, that is 61.5%. It should be noted that all the amino acids involved in binding to sugars at the 1α site are conserved in kirkiin and ricin, while at the 2γ site, Glu235 and His246 in kirkiin change to Ala237 and Tyr248 in ricin, respectively (Figure 3). These changes could explain the large differences in lactose and D-galactose affinities between kirkiin and stenodactylin and ricin (Table 1). In fact, the affinity of ricin for D-galactose is four and eight times higher than those of kirkiin and stenodactylin, respectively, and the affinity of ricin for lactose is 16 times greater than that of kirkiin or stenodactylin.

This prompted us to study how D-galactose binds to kirkiin 1α and 2γ sites in comparison to ricin, since glucose does not bind to kirkiin, and therefore, lactose has to bind to this protein via galactose as with ricin. For this purpose, we perform a comparative molecular docking study using Autodock 4.2. Using the sequence of the kirkiin B chain where the first nine amino acids, corresponding to subdomain 1λ were excluded, a structure was obtained by comparative modeling in the I-Tasser server that presented better values of C-score (1.32), Tm score (0.90 $\pm$ 0.06), and RMSD (3.2 $\pm$ 2.2 Å) than the model obtained with the whole protein. Docking was performed with D-galactose and lactose, and solutions matching the two structures were chosen. As shown in Figure S2, with the 1α site of ricin, there are no differences between the results obtained by molecular docking with D-galactose or lactose and those obtained by crystallography and X-ray diffraction, while small differences are observed at the 2γ site, although the orientation of the pyranosic ring is identical.

As shown in Figure 5, the amino acids involved in D-galactose binding at the 1α site of ricin are conserved in kirkiin, and the way D-galactose binds is very similar in both proteins. In both cases, the binding of β-D-galactopyranose is the result of the C–H–π interaction between the aromatic ring of Trp37 and the apolar face of the pyranosic ring of galactose. The polar groups of the polar face of galactose form hydrogen bonds with the amino acids Asp22, Asp25, Gln35, and Asn46, and, in the case of kirkiin, the hydrogen bonds can also be formed with Lys24 and Lys40. In snake gourd seed lectin (SGLS), a non-toxic type 2 RIP obtained from seeds of *Trichosanthes cucumerina* L. (= *Trichosanthes anguina* L.), the apolar face of the pyranosic ring of galactose binds to the aromatic ring of Tyr36, while the polar face forms hydrogen bonds with the amino acids on the other side of the pocket of the 1α site, mainly with Gly24 [24] (Figure 5).

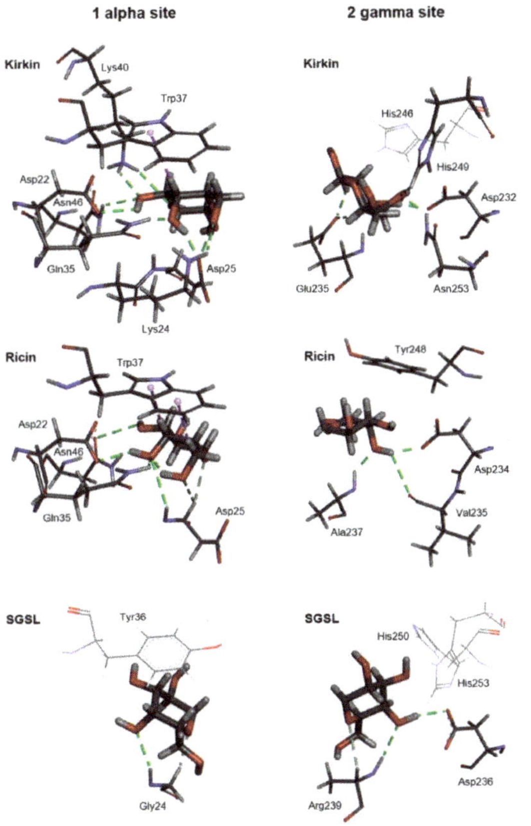

Figure 5. Three-dimensional models of the galactose-binding sites from kirkiin, ricin, and SGSL. The galactose-binding sites from either kirkiin, ricin (PDB 2AAI), and SGSL (PDB 5Y97) complexed with β-D-galactopyranose (thick sticks) are represented. The amino acids that bind the galactose molecule by either C–H–π interactions (dashed purple lines) or both conventional (dashed green lines) and non-conventional (dashed light green lines) hydrogen bonds are represented by thin sticks. His246 from kirkiin, and Tyr36, His250, and His253 from SGSL are also represented (lines).

Unlike the 1α site, the 2γ site of kirkiin is very different from that of ricin. In ricin, the aromatic ring of Tyr248 is oriented toward the apolar face of the pyranosic ring, being able to establish a C–H–π interaction with the apolar face of it. The polar face of D-galactopyranose establishes hydrogen bonds, on the other side of the pocket of the 2γ site, with the amino acids Asp234, Val235, and Ala237 (Figure 5). In kirkiin (as in stenodactylin), Tyr248 is replaced by His246. Unlike ricin, the apolar face of galactose is not oriented toward the aromatic ring and there can be no C–H–π interaction between galactose and histidine. The binding is reached by hydrogen bonds with Asp232, Glu235, His249, and Asn253. This arrangement is similar to that presented at the 2γ site of the SGSL, where the apolar face is not oriented toward His250, and the polar face forms hydrogen bonds with Asp236 and Arg239 (Figure 5).

3. Discussion

Kirkiin, a type 2 RIP isolated from *A. kirkii* caudex, is one of the most potent plant toxins known, with a cytotoxicity comparable to that of stenodactylin and ricin [8]. The aim of the present work was to determine the complete amino acid sequence of kirkiin as well as to predict the protein structure by using computational homology modeling.

Sequence analysis showed that kirkiin is encoded by a 1572 bp gene without introns, as previously reported for other RIPs, such as volkensin [13], ricin [25], abrin [26], and viscumin [27]. Kirkiin shares a high degree of identity with the type 2 RIPs stenodactylin and volkensin, since all toxins are phylogenetically related. This expected high identity also explains why kirkiin highly cross-reacted with serum against stenodactylin and volkensin [8]. The N-terminal sequences of kirkiin A and B chains were found to be identical to those of stenodactylin, with the exception of the residue Phe in position 7 in the stenodactylin A chain, which is replaced by Leu in kirkiin A chain. This substitution is also present in the A chains of modeccin and the isoform 1 of lanceolin. Interestingly, the N-terminal sequence of kirkiin A chain shares the presence of an additional cysteine residue with the A chains of other *Adenia* RIPs, except for volkensin. It could be of interest to better investigate in the future the role of this cysteine residue, since the reduction of the disulfide bridge inside the cell is important for type 2 RIP toxicity.

The complete amino acid sequence showed that kirkiin, similar to stenodactylin, contains the highest number of cysteine residues among type 2 RIPs. It is known for the type 2 RIPs that the C-terminal cysteine of the A chain forms an interchain disulfide bridge with the cysteine at the B chain N-terminus [28]. Similarly, Cys246 of the kirkiin A chain is involved in a disulfide bridge with Cys4 of the B chain. The type 2 RIP B chain consists of two lectin domains, each organized around two disulfide bridges [29]. This scheme is also present in kirkiin (Cys20 to Cys39 and Cys63 to Cys78 for lectin 1 of B chain; Cys149 to Cys162 and Cys188 to Cys206 for lectin 2 of B chain). Three other cysteine residues are included in the kirkiin B chain (Cys59, Cys191, and Cys195). In the 3D model, Cys59 seems to be isolated in lectin 1, while Cys191 and Cys195 are located in a loop in lectin 2, which is close enough to form a disulfide bridge. This pattern was already observed in the volkensin 3D model [13]; however, the role of these cysteine residues is still unknown.

Two glycosylation sites are located in the kirkiin B chain. The presence of carbohydrates could explain the difference in the molecular weight of the B chain determined on the basis of the amino acid sequence (28.5 kDa) and on that observed by electrophoretic mobility (35 kDa) [8]. The glycosylation level of RIPs has proven to be important in explaining their toxic activity. It can influence the protein structure, impacting either the overall structure or the local conformation, and consequently, it can affect RIP intracellular transport to the endoplasmic reticulum and to other compartments, thus influencing its cytotoxicity [30,31].

A molecular model of kirkiin has been elaborated on the basis of the crystallographic coordinates of ricin, which shares a high sequence homology with kirkiin. Knowledge about the amino acid sequence associated with the structure analysis of the RIP is essential to understand the protein function and to correlate structural differences to the cytotoxic mechanisms of RIPs. The three-dimensional model obtained for kirkiin revealed that it shares the general structure of type 2 RIPs. The amino acids of the active site, responsible for the enzymatic mechanism of RIPs [32], are also conserved in kirkiin: Tyr74, Tyr113, and Trp200 are the amino acids directly involved in substrate binding, whereas Glu163 and Arg166 are the amino acids responsible for the catalysis. The highly conserved Phe167 located in the active site is also present in kirkiin; its function is still unclear but seems to be involved in stabilizing the conformation of the side chain of Arg166 [33]. Most of the additional residues participating in the active site of ricin (Asn78, Arg134, Gln173, Ala178, Glu208, and Asn209) are also conserved in kirkiin. They are involved in the stabilization of the active site, and almost all are conserved among the A chains of type 2 RIPs [34,35]. Most of these amino acids are conserved in the kirkiin A chain (Asn72, Arg123, and Ala164), except for Gln173, Glu208, and Asn209 in ricin that are replaced in kirkiin by Gly159, Val197, and Thr198, respectively. These substitutions are also present in the stenodactylin [22] and volkensin A chains [13]. In addition, Ser204, located close to the active site and evolutionarily conserved among RIPs with the function of stabilizing the conformation of the side chain of Trp200 [36], is also conserved in kirkiin. Almost all the amino acids involved in sugar binding in the 1α and 2γ subdomains of the ricin B chain [37] are conserved in kirkiin (Asp22, Asp25, Gln35, and Trp37 for the 1α subdomain and Asp232, Ile244, Asn253, and Gln254 for the 2γ subdomain). Two exceptions in the 2γ subdomain were identified for Ala237 and Tyr248 in ricin, which are replaced with Glu235 and His246 in kirkiin, respectively. The same substitutions were observed in stenodactylin [22] and volkensin [13]. In particular, the presence of His instead of Tyr was also identified in *R. communis* agglutinin [38] and in PMRIPm of *Polygonatum multiflorum* [35]. A previous study demonstrated that the substitution of Tyr248 with His in the ricin B chain introduced a positive charge in the 2γ subdomain, preventing the interaction between the pyranose ring of galactose and the aromatic ring of Tyr. This change caused a reduction in the binding activity of ricin [39]. Moreover, the presence of the aromatic residue Phe249 in ebulin l from *Sambucus ebulus*, instead of Tyr248 in ricin, results in a deficient sugar binding and a consequently lower RIP cytotoxicity [40]. These data suggest that the sugar affinity is essential to explain the biological activity of RIPs. The recognition and binding to exposed galactose residues on cell membrane is the first step in RIP–cell interaction. Thus, small differences in sugar binding might affect RIP cytotoxic activity. Most of the RIPs have galactose/N-acetylgalactosamine (gal/galNAc) affinity, but some of them can also show different sugar specificity. For example, *Sambucus nigra* agglutinin I has affinity for both gal/galNAc and sialic acid [41]. Mistletoe lectin I has specificity for galactose, L-arabinose, and poor affinity for sialic acid [42]. Changes in the 2γ subdomain of the *Sambucus* tetrameric RIPs (Glu235 by Gln, His246 by Tyr, and His249 by Thr or Asn) cause specificity toward galactose and N-acetyl neuraminic acid [43]. Moreover, changes in both 1α and 2γ binding sites of *Iris hollandica* RIPs (Trp37 by Ser and His246 by Trp) are responsible for specificity toward mannose [44]. In the case of kirkiin, the hypothesis that changes in the 2γ site could affect cell binding does not correlate with the high cytotoxicity that kirkiin has shown in previous studies [8]. For this reason, we considered it interesting to study the sugar affinity properties of kirkiin in order to have more detailed information that would help us understand its unique properties. Hemagglutination inhibition assay showed that kirkiin and stenodactylin have similar affinities for D-galactose and lactose (Table 1), which is probably due to the high sequence identity of the sugar binding sites. Nevertheless, the affinity of kirkiin for these sugars was lower with respect to ricin. According to docking experiments, both the 1α and 2γ sites of kirkiin can bind lactose and D-galactose. The 1α sites of both ricin and kirkiin are identical. The interaction of tryptophan with the apolar face of D-galactopyranose allows the formation of numerous hydrogen bonds between the polar face and the amino acids on the other side of the 1α site pocket. It is worth noting that the orientation of the C-4 hydroxyl group of D-glucopyranose toward the aromatic rings would prevent this type of binding. In SGSL, the binding to the 1α site is very different [24]. The lack of toxicity of SGLS has been attributed to the result of a combination of changes in the active site of the A chain (it does not bind adenine) and the sugar binding sites of the B chain. In SGLS, the aromatic ring of Tyr36 could play the same role as tryptophan in kirkiin and ricin, and the polar face of the pyranosic ring could form hydrogen bonds with the amino acids on the other side of the pocket of the 1α site, mainly with Gly24 (Figure 5), but also with other amino acids. However, this binding would be weak, and for this reason, the 1α site can bind D-galactose but cannot retain it [24].

Since the kirkiin 1α site is identical to that of ricin, the two amino acid substitutions in the 2γ site, in particular the replacement of Tyr248 of ricin with His246, are evidently sufficient to lower the affinity of kirkiin for these sugars. These changes cause a different arrangement within the pocket of the 2γ site with respect to ricin, which could justify the low affinity for lactose and D-galactose. This arrangement is similar to that of the 2γ site of SGSL, which is able to bind and retain galactose [24].

All these data show that kirkiin has a high degree of identity with RIPs from *Adenia* genus plants as well as a structure that preserves the overall folding of type 2 RIPs.

Despite the substantial difference in the structure of the 2γ site with respect to ricin that may explain the lower affinity for sugars, kirkiin and *Adenia* RIPs are the most toxic plant proteins [8]. Therefore, their biological properties, especially cytotoxicity, could be correlated to other mechanisms that overcome the differences in cell binding. The high cytotoxic potential of kirkiin and its ability to elicit different cell death pathways makes kirkiin a suitable candidate as a pharmacological tool for drug targeting. The high toxicity of native kirkiin would allow its use only for loco-regional treatments. However, the kirkiin A chain could be linked to carriers targeting cancer cells in systemic therapy. Further studies will be useful to better clarify the modalities and the types of triggered cell death and the consequent biological behavior of kirkiin in vivo.

4. Materials and Methods

4.1. Materials

Kirkiin was purified from the caudex of *Adenia kirkii* as described by Bortolotti et al. [8]. *Adenia* plants volkensin and stenodactylin were purchased from Exotica Botanical Rarities, Erkelenz-Golkrath, Germany, while *A. kirkii* was purchased from Mbuyu–Sukkulenten, Bielefeld, Germany. If not used immediately on arrival, the plants were kept in the greenhouse of the Botanical Garden of the University of Bologna.

Genomic DNA from *A. kirkii* was extracted through DNeasy Minikit (Qiagen Iberia SL, Barcelona, Spain). Primers were synthesized by Integrated DNA Technologies (Leuven, Belgium). Taq Polymerase was obtained from Biotools B&M Labs S.A. (Madrid, Spain). PCR products were purified using the NucleoSpin® Gel and PCR Clean-up kit (Macherey-Nagel GmbH & Co KG, Düren, Germany). Molecular cloning of PCR products was carried out using TA Cloning® Kit Dual Promoter (Invitrogen-Thermo Fisher Scientific, Alcobendas, Spain). Plasmids were sequenced by CENIT Support system (Villamayor, Salamanca, Spain).

4.2. Methods

4.2.1. Isolation of DNA

The caudex of *A. kirkii* was disrupted using a mortar and pestle and grinded to a fine powder under liquid nitrogen and total DNA was extracted through DNeasy Minikit (Qiagen), according to the manufacturer's instruction. Then, 1.2 μg of total DNA was obtained from 100 mg of frozen tissue. The DNA content was determined by a Beckman DU 640 Spectrophotometer (Beckman, Brea, CA, USA).

4.2.2. Primer Design for PCR Amplification

Gene-specific primers for the full-length kirkiin sequence were designed and synthesized based on volkensin and stenodactylin amino acid sequences (CAD61022 and MT580807) and N-terminal sequences available for *Adenia* RIPs. Four oligonucleotides were designed for PCR amplification of the kirkiin gene: A2 for N-terminal sequence of the A chain; B1 and B1 reverse (B1R) for N-terminal sequence of the B chain, and B5 reverse (B5R) for the C-terminal end of the B chain. The sequences of the primers are reported in Table 2.

Table 2. Primer sequences.

Primer	Sequence
A2	5′ GCCACGGTAGAGAGRTACACT 3′
B1R	5′ AAGTCGTCTCCCCGGAAGGGC 3′
B1	5′ TGCCCTTCCGGGGAGACGACT 3′
B5R	5′ TAGGAACCATTGCTGGTTGGA 3′

4.2.3. Amino Acid Sequencing by Edman Degradation

Kirkiin was blotted both in reduced and non-reduced form onto PVDF membrane (Immobilon P membrane) in 50 mM sodium borate, pH 9.0/20% methanol/0.1% SDS at 1 mA/cm^2 PVDF membrane for 2–3 h at 4 °C. The protein band was stained by Ponceau Red (0.5% Ponceau S, 1% acetic acid in Milli-Q water). The blotted bands that corresponded to kirkiin A and B chains (50 µg each) were cut and directly subjected to N-terminal automated protein sequencing using the PPSQ–33B sequencer (Shimadzu Corporation, Tokyo, Japan). Edman degradation was performed by Protein and Peptide Sequencing Service—Institute of Biosciences and Bioresources (National Research Council, Naples).

4.2.4. Gene Amplification and Cloning

Genomic DNA was used as a template for PCR amplification in order to determine the amino acid sequence of kirkiin. PCR was conducted using the thermal cycler Gene Amp PCR system 2400 (Perkin Elmer, Waltham, MA, USA). The PCR reaction for gene amplification included 40 ng of total DNA, 0.5 µM of each primer, PCR buffer/Mg^{2+} (Tris HCl 75 mM pH 9.0, KCl 50 mM, $(NH_4)_2SO_4$ 20 mM, $MgCl_2$ 2 mM), 0.25 mM dNTPs Mix, and 0.5 U/µL Taq Polymerase (Biotools). PCR amplification was carried out with the following conditions: an initial denaturation at 94 °C for 3 min, followed by 40 cycles of 94 °C for 30 s, 55 °C for 45 s, and 72 °C for 2 min. Three couples of primers were used to detect the full-length amino acid sequence of kirkiin (A2–B1R for the A chain and part of the B chain, B1–B5R for the B chain; A2–B5R for the complete sequence). The amplified fragments were analyzed by agarose gel electrophoresis, showing the expected size of about 0.8 kb for the A chain with part of the B chain (Figure S1A) and about 1.6 kb for the entire sequence (Figure S1B). B1–B5R failed to amplify the target region. PCR products were purified using the NucleoSpin® Gel and PCR Clean-up kit (Macherey-Nagel), according to the manufacturer's instruction. The two purified amplicons were ligated into the pCR®II vector (TA Cloning® Kit Dual Promoter, Invitrogen) and then were used to transform the highly competent *E. coli* InVαF′ cells. The purified plasmids were sequenced by CENIT Support system. The information obtained on the sequence was analyzed using the algorithms available on http://expasy.org (accessed on 15 October 2021) [11].

4.2.5. Sequence Retrieval and Alignment

The sequences of stenodactylin (Accession number MT580807) and volkensin (Accession number Q70US9) are available in the National Center for Biotechnology Information (NCBI) sequence database (https://www.ncbi.nlm.nih.gov/protein/ (accessed on 15 October 2021)). Sequence alignment was performed using the Clustal Omega server (https://www.ebi.ac.uk/Tools/msa/clustalo/ (accessed on 15 October 2021)) [16]. Glycosylation sites were predicted using the NetNGlyc1.0 server [18].

4.2.6. Protein Structure Studies and Graphical Representation

The structures of ricin (accession numbers 2AAI, 3RTI, and 3RTJ) and SGSL (accession number 5Y97) are available in the Protein Data Bank (https://www.rcsb.org/ (accessed on 15 October 2021)). Three-dimensional structural modeling of kirkiin was carried out on the I-TASSER server (https://zhanglab.ccmb.med.umich.edu/I-TASSER/ (accessed on 15 October 2021)) [45]. Study and graph representations of protein structures were performed with the aid of the Discovery Studio Visualizer suite (v16.1.0) (https://www.3dsbiovia.com/ (accessed on 15 October 2021)).

4.2.7. Hemagglutination Activity and Carbohydrate-Binding Properties

Hemagglutination activity (HA) was assayed using 2% human erythrocyte suspension collected from voluntary donors (0+, A+, and B+). Blood samples were collected in phosphate-buffered saline (PBS) and centrifuged at 500× *g*. The erythrocyte pellet was washed and resuspended in the same buffer to make 2% red blood cell suspension. The HA was determined in microtiter plates. Each well contained 50 µL of serial dilutions of the proteins and 50 μL of erythrocyte suspension and the plates were incubated for 1 h at room temperature. The minimum concentration of protein causing complete agglutination was visually evaluated. For hemagglutination inhibition assay, ten sugars (D-glucose 3.2 M, D-galactose 1.5 M, D-Fructose 3.2 M, D-Mannose 3.0 M, D-Sorbitol 2.9 M, D-Mannitol 0.9 M, L-Fucose 1.1 M, N-Acetyl-D-mannosamine 6.8 M, Lactose 0.7 M, Sucrose 1.2 M) were tested for their ability to inhibit the HA of the RIPs with 0+ blood group. Each well contained 25 μL of carbohydrates serially diluted and an equal volume of the RIP at a concentration one titer higher than the HA dose. An equal volume of erythrocyte suspension (50 μL) was added to each well and incubated for 1 h at room temperature. The maximum concentration of the tested sugars that completely inhibited HA activity was determined.

4.2.8. Molecular Docking

The structures of beta-D-galactose (PubChem CID 439353) and beta-lactose (PubChem CID 6134) are available in the PubChem database (https://pubchem.ncbi.nlm.nih.gov/ (accessed on 15 October 2021)) [46]. Docking was carried out using Autodock 4.2 (http://autodock.scripps.edu/ (accessed on 15 October 2021)), as previously described [47]. Docking of D-galactose was performed on a grid of 120 × 120 × 120 points, with the addition of a central grid point. The grid was centered on the C4 of the galactose of either the 1α site or the 2γ site of the 2AAI ricin structure. Grid spacing was 0.125 Angstroms, leading to a grid of 15 × 15 × 15 Angstroms. For each molecule, 100 docking runs were performed. The generated 100 docking poses were clustered by root mean square (RMS) difference with a cutoff value of 0.5 Angstroms for each case. The top-ranked pose of the most populated clusters was retained and further analyzed with the Discovery Studio Visualizer suite (v16.1.0). The docking of beta-lactose was performed as indicated for D-galactose but using a grid of 124 × 124 × 124 points and a grid spacing of 0.180 Angstroms, leading to a grid of 22.32 × 22.32 × 22.32 Angstroms. The generated 100 docking poses were clustered by RMS difference with a cutoff value 2.0 Angstroms for each case. The top-ranked pose of the most populated clusters was retained and further analyzed with the Discovery Studio Visualizer suite (v16.1.0). Finally, the results obtained with D-galactose and beta-lactose were matched, and the coinciding solutions were selected.

5. Conclusions

The knowledge of amino acid sequence and the 3D structure prediction of kirkiin represent essential tools because of the potential use of kirkiin in medicine, for cancer treatment, and of its biotechnological applications in neuroscience. Moreover, the comparison between the structural properties of kirkiin and those of other type 2 RIPs is useful for explaining the differences in enzymatic activity and toxicity.

Supplementary Materials: The following are available online at https://www.mdpi.com/article/10.3390/toxins13120862/s1: Figure S1: Amplification of kirkiin A chain with part of the B chain (A, lane 1), and the entire sequence (B, lane 1). Mw: λ Hind III/EcoRI double digest DNA marker. The red squares indicate the amplification products. Figure S2: Comparison of the three-dimensional models of ricin (PDB 2AAI) sugar-binding sites 1 alpha (left) and 2 gamma (right) bound to D-galactose. The results obtained using AutoDock 4.2 with either β-D-galactopyranose (green lines, PubChem CID 439353) and β-lactose (blue lines, PubChem CID 6134) are compared with those obtained by X-ray diffraction (gray lines) as reported previously [48]. The amino acids of the sugar-binding sites are represented by sticks. In the case of β-lactose, only the galactose part is represented.

Author Contributions: Conceptualization, R.I., J.M.F., A.B. and L.P.; methodology and validation, R.I., S.M. and J.M.F.; formal analysis and investigation, M.B., S.M. and L.C.; all the authors participated to write, review and edit the manuscript; funding acquisition, A.B., L.P. and J.M.F. All authors have read and agreed to the published version of the manuscript.

Funding: This work was supported by funds for selected research topics from the Alma Mater Studiorum, University of Bologna and by the Pallotti Legacies for Cancer Research; Fondazione CARISBO, Project 2019.0539; Grant VA033G19 (Consejería de Educación, Junta de Castilla y León) to the GIR ProtIBio.

Institutional Review Board Statement: Not applicable.

Informed Consent Statement: Not applicable.

Data Availability Statement: The DNA sequence for kirkiin was submitted to GenBank (accession number: OK283399).

Conflicts of Interest: The authors declare no conflict of interest.

References

1. Polito, L.; Bortolotti, M.; Maiello, S.; Battelli, M.G.; Bolognesi, A. Plants Producing Ribosome-Inactivating Proteins in Traditional Medicine. *Molecules* **2016**, *21*, 1560. [CrossRef]
2. Bortolotti, M.; Mercatelli, D.; Polito, L. *Momordica charantia*, a Nutraceutical Approach for Inflammatory Related Diseases. *Front. Pharmacol.* **2019**, *10*, 486. [CrossRef]
3. Battelli, M.G.; Barbieri, L.; Bolognesi, A.; Buonamici, L.; Valbonesi, P.; Polito, L.; Van Damme, E.J.; Peumans, W.J.; Stirpe, F. Ribosome-inactivating lectins with polynucleotide: Adenosine glycosidase activity. *FEBS Lett.* **1997**, *408*, 355–359. [CrossRef]
4. Pelosi, E.; Lubelli, C.; Polito, L.; Barbieri, L.; Bolognesi, A.; Stirpe, F. Ribosome-inactivating proteins and other lectins from Adenia (Passifloraceae). *Toxicon* **2005**, *46*, 658–663. [CrossRef] [PubMed]
5. Monti, B.; D'Alessandro, C.; Farini, V.; Bolognesi, A.; Polazzi, E.; Contestabile, A.; Stirpe, F.; Battelli, M.G. In vitro and in vivo toxicity of type 2 ribosome-inactivating proteins lanceolin and stenodactylin on glial and neuronal cells. *Neurotoxicology* **2007**, *28*, 637–644. [CrossRef]
6. Polito, L.; Bortolotti, M.; Pedrazzi, M.; Mercatelli, D.; Battelli, M.G.; Bolognesi, A. Apoptosis and necroptosis induced by stenodactylin in neuroblastoma cells can be completely prevented through caspase inhibition plus catalase or necrostatin-1. *Phytomedicine* **2016**, *23*, 32–41. [CrossRef] [PubMed]
7. Mercatelli, D.; Bortolotti, M.; Andresen, V.; Sulen, A.; Polito, L.; Gjertsen, B.T.; Bolognesi, A. Early response to the plant toxin stenodactylin in acute myeloid leukemia cells involves inflammatory and apoptotic signaling. *Front. Pharmacol.* **2020**, *11*, 630. [CrossRef]
8. Bortolotti, M.; Maiello, S.; Ferreras, J.M.; Iglesias, R.; Polito, L.; Bolognesi, A. Kirkiin: A New Toxic Type 2 Ribosome-Inactivating Protein from the Caudex of *Adenia kirkii*. *Toxins* **2021**, *13*, 81. [CrossRef]
9. Polito, L.; Djemil, A.; Bortolotti, M. Plant Toxin-Based Immunotoxins for Cancer Therapy: A Short Overview. *Biomedicines* **2016**, *4*, 12. [CrossRef]
10. Polito, L.; Mercatelli, D.; Bortolotti, M.; Maiello, S.; Djemil, A.; Battelli, M.G.; Bolognesi, A. Two Saporin-Containing Immunotoxins Specific for CD20 and CD22 Show Different Behavior in Killing Lymphoma Cells. *Toxins* **2017**, *9*, 182. [CrossRef] [PubMed]
11. ExPASy Bioinformatics Resource Portal. Available online: https://www.expasy.org/ (accessed on 15 October 2021).
12. Montecucchi, P.C.; Lazzarini, A.M.; Barbieri, L.; Stirpe, F.; Soria, M.; Lappi, D. N-terminal sequence of some ribosome-inactivating proteins. *Int. J. Pept. Protein Res.* **1989**, *33*, 263–267. [CrossRef]
13. Chambery, A.; Di Maro, A.; Monti, M.M.; Stirpe, F.; Parente, A. Volkensin from *Adenia volkensii* Harms (kilyambiti plant), a type 2 ribosome-inactivating protein. *Eur. J. Biochem.* **2004**, *271*, 108–117. [CrossRef] [PubMed]
14. Stirpe, F.; Bolognesi, A.; Bortolotti, M.; Farini, V.; Lubelli, C.; Pelosi, E.; Polito, L.; Dozza, B.; Strocchi, P.; Chambery, A.; et al. Characterization of highly toxic type 2 ribosome-inactivating proteins from *Adenia lanceolata* and *Adenia stenodactyla* (Passifloraceae). *Toxicon* **2007**, *50*, 94–105. [CrossRef]
15. Sievers, F.; Wilm, A.; Dineen, D.; Gibson, T.J.; Karplus, K.; Li, W.; Lopez, R.; McWilliam, H.; Remmert, M.; Söding, J.; et al. Fast, scalable generation of high-quality protein multiple sequence alignments using Clustal Omega. *Mol. Syst. Biol.* **2011**, *7*, 539. [CrossRef] [PubMed]
16. Polito, L.; Bortolotti, M.; Battelli, M.G.; Calafato, G.; Bolognesi, A. Ricin: An Ancient Story for a Timeless Plant Toxin. *Toxins* **2019**, *11*, 324. [CrossRef]
17. Lappi, D.A.; Kapmeyer, W.; Beglau, J.M.; Kaplan, N.O. The disulfide bond connecting the chains of ricin. *Proc. Natl. Acad. Sci. USA* **1978**, *75*, 1096–1100. [CrossRef]
18. NetNGlyc 1.0 Server. Available online: http://www.cbs.dtu.dk/services/NetNGlyc/ (accessed on 15 October 2021).
19. Reyes, L.F.; Nobre, T.M.; Pavinatto, F.J.; Zaniquelli, M.E.; Caseli, L.; Oliveira, O.N., Jr.; Araujo, A.P. The role of the C-terminal region of pulchellin A-chain in the interaction with membrane model systems. *Biochim. Biophys. Acta* **2012**, *1818*, 82–89. [CrossRef]
20. Baykal, U.; Tumer, N.E. The C-terminus of pokeweed antiviral protein has distinct roles in transport to the cytosol, ribosome depurination and cytotoxicity. *Plant J.* **2007**, *49*, 995–1007. [CrossRef] [PubMed]
21. Villafranca, J.E.; Robertus, J.D. Ricin B chain is a product of gene duplication. *J. Biol. Chem.* **1981**, *256*, 554–556. [CrossRef]
22. Iglesias, R.; Polito, L.; Bortolotti, M.; Pedrazzi, M.; Citores, L.; Ferreras, J.M.; Bolognesi, A. Primary Sequence and 3D Structure Prediction of the Plant Toxin Stenodactylin. *Toxins* **2020**, *12*, 538. [CrossRef]

23. Nicolson, G.L.; Blaustein, J.; Etzler, M.E. Characterization of two plant lectins from *Ricinus communis* and their quantitative interaction with a murine lymphoma. *Biochemistry* **1974**, *13*, 196–204. [CrossRef] [PubMed]
24. Chandran, T.; Sivaji, N.; Surolia, A.; Vijayan, M. Ligand binding and retention in snake gourd seed lectin (SGSL). A crystallographic, thermodynamic and molecular dynamics study. *Glycobiology* **2018**, *28*, 968–977. [CrossRef]
25. Halling, K.C.; Halling, A.C.; Murray, E.E.; Ladin, B.F.; Houston, L.L.; Weaver, R.F. Genomic cloning and characterization of a ricin gene from *Ricinus communis*. *Nucleic Acids Res.* **1985**, *13*, 8019–8033. [CrossRef] [PubMed]
26. Evensen, G.; Mathiesen, A.; Sundan, A. Direct molecular cloning and expression of two distinct abrin A-chains. *J. Biol. Chem.* **1991**, *266*, 6848–6852. [CrossRef]
27. Eck, J.; Langer, M.; Mockel, B.; Baur, A.; Rothe, M.; Zinke, H.; Lentzen, H. Cloning of the mistletoe lectin gene and characterisation of the recombinant A-chain. *Eur. J. Biochem.* **1999**, *264*, 775–784. [CrossRef] [PubMed]
28. Robertus, J.D.; Monzingo, A.F. The structure of ribosome inactivating proteins. *Mini Rev. Med. Chem.* **2004**, *4*, 477–486. [CrossRef]
29. Montfort, W.; Villafranca, J.E.; Monzingo, A.F.; Ernst, S.R.; Katzin, B.; Rutenber, E.; Xuong, N.H.; Hamlin, R.; Robertus, J.D. The three-dimensional structure of ricin at 2.8 A. *J. Biol. Chem.* **1987**, *262*, 5398–5403. [CrossRef]
30. Liu, W.Y. Research on ribosome-inactivating proteins from angiospermae to gymnospermae and cryptogamia. *Am. J. Transl. Res.* **2017**, *9*, 5719–5742. [PubMed]
31. Sehgal, P.; Kumar, O.; Kameswararao, M.; Ravindran, J.; Khan, M.; Sharma, S.; Vijayaraghavan, R.; Prasad, G.B.K.S. Differential toxicity profile of ricin isoforms correlates with their glycosylation levels. *Toxicology* **2011**, *282*, 56–67. [CrossRef]
32. De Virgilio, M.; Lombardi, A.; Caliandro, R.; Fabbrini, M.S. Ribosome-inactivating proteins: From plant defense to tumor attack. *Toxins* **2010**, *2*, 2699–2737. [CrossRef]
33. Di Maro, A.; Citores, L.; Russo, R.; Iglesias, R.; Ferreras, J.M. Sequence comparison and phylogenetic analysis by the Maximum Likelihood method of ribosome-inactivating proteins from angiosperms. *Plant Mol. Biol.* **2014**, *85*, 575–588. [CrossRef]
34. Katzin, B.J.; Collins, E.J.; Robertus, J.D. Structure of ricin A-chain at 2.5 A. *Proteins* **1991**, *10*, 251–259. [CrossRef]
35. Van Damme, E.J.; Hao, Q.; Charels, D.; Barre, A.; Rougé, P.; Van Leuven, F.; Peumans, W.J. Characterization and molecular cloning of two different type 2 ribosome-inactivating proteins from the monocotyledonous plant *Polygonatum multiflorum*. *Eur. J. Biochem.* **2000**, *267*, 2746–2759. [CrossRef] [PubMed]
36. Chambery, A.; Pisante, M.; Di Maro, A.; Di Zazzo, E.; Ruvo, M.; Costantini, S.; Colonna, G.; Parente, A. Invariant Ser211 is involved in the catalysis of PD-L4, type I RIP from *Phytolacca dioica* leaves. *Proteins* **2007**, *67*, 209–218. [CrossRef]
37. Shi, W.W.; Mak, A.N.; Wong, K.B.; Shaw, P.C. Structures and Ribosomal Interaction of Ribosome-Inactivating Proteins. *Molecules* **2016**, *21*, 1588. [CrossRef]
38. Roberts, L.M.; Lamb, F.I.; Pappin, D.J.; Lord, J.M. The primary sequence of *Ricinus communis* agglutinin. Comparison with ricin. *J. Biol. Chem.* **1985**, *260*, 15682–15686. [CrossRef]
39. Lehar, S.M.; Pedersen, J.T.; Kamath, R.S.; Swimmer, C.; Goldmacher, V.S.; Lambert, J.M.; Blättler, W.A.; Guild, B.C. Mutational and structural analysis of the lectin activity in binding domain 2 of ricin B chain. *Protein Eng.* **1994**, *7*, 1261–1266. [CrossRef]
40. Ferreras, J.M.; Citores, L.; Iglesias, R.; Jiménez, P.; Girbés, T. Sambucus Ribosome-Inactivating Proteins and Lectins. Toxic Plant Proteins. In *Toxic Plant Proteins–Plant Cell Monographs*, 1st ed.; Lord, J.M., Hartley, M.R., Eds.; Springer: Berlin/Heidelberg, Germany, 2010; Volume 18, pp. 107–131.
41. Van Damme, E.J.; Roy, S.; Barre, A.; Citores, L.; Mostafapous, K.; Rougé, P.; Van Leuven, F.; Girbés, T.; Goldstein, I.J.; Peumans, W.J. Elderberry (Sambucus nigra) bark contains two structurally different Neu5Ac(alpha2,6)Gal/GalNAc-binding type 2 ribosome-inactivating proteins. *Eur. J. Biochem.* **1997**, *245*, 648–655. [CrossRef]
42. Mishra, V.; Sharma, R.S.; Yadav, S.; Babu, C.R.; Singh, T.P. Purification and characterization of four isoforms of Himalayan mistletoe ribosome-inactivating protein from Viscum album having unique sugar affinity. *Arch. Biochem. Biophys.* **2004**, *423*, 288–301. [CrossRef] [PubMed]
43. Iglesias, R.; Ferreras, J.M.; Di Maro, A.; Citores, L. Ebulin-RP, a novel member of the Ebulin gene family with low cytotoxicity as a result of deficient sugar binding domains. *Biochim. Biophys. Acta Gen. Subj.* **2018**, *1862*, 460–473. [CrossRef]
44. Hao, Q.; Van Damme, E.J.; Hause, B.; Barre, A.; Chen, Y.; Rougé, P.; Peumans, W.J. Iris bulbs express type 1 and type 2 ribosome-inactivating proteins with unusual properties. *Plant Physiol.* **2001**, *125*, 866–876. [CrossRef]
45. Yang, J.; Zhang, Y. I-TASSER server: New development for protein structure and function predictions. *Nucleic Acids Res.* **2015**, *43*, W174–W181. [CrossRef] [PubMed]
46. Kim, S.; Chen, J.; Cheng, T.; Gindulyte, A.; He, J.; He, S.; Li, Q.; Shoemaker, B.A.; Thiessen, P.A.; Yu, B.; et al. PubChem in 2021: New data content and improved web interfaces. *Nucleic Acids Res.* **2021**, *49*, D1388–D1395. [CrossRef]
47. Morris, G.M.; Huey, R.; Lindstrom, W.; Sanner, M.F.; Belew, R.K.; Goodsell, D.S.; Olson, A.J. AutoDock4 and AutoDockTools4: Automated docking with selective receptor flexibility. *J. Comput. Chem.* **2009**, *30*, 2785–2791. [CrossRef] [PubMed]
48. Rutenber, E.; Robertus, J.D. Structure of ricin B-chain at 2.5 A resolution. *Proteins* **1991**, *10*, 260–269. [CrossRef] [PubMed]

MDPI
St. Alban-Anlage 66
4052 Basel
Switzerland
Tel. +41 61 683 77 34
Fax +41 61 302 89 18
www.mdpi.com

Toxins Editorial Office
E-mail: toxins@mdpi.com
www.mdpi.com/journal/toxins

www.ingramcontent.com/pod-product-compliance
Lightning Source LLC
LaVergne TN
LVHW070551100526
838202LV00012B/439
9783036530642